Evaluating Managed Mental Health Services

The Fort Bragg Experiment

Evaluating Managed Mental Health Services

The Fort Bragg Experiment

**Leonard Bickman, Pamela R. Guthrie,
E. Michael Foster, E. Warren Lambert,
Wm. Thomas Summerfelt,
Carolyn S. Breda, and
Craig Anne Heflinger**

*Vanderbilt University
Nashville, Tennessee*

PLENUM PRESS • NEW YORK AND LONDON

Library of Congress Cataloging-in-Publication Data

ISBN 0306450445
ISBN 0306484374

© 1995 Plenum Press, New York
A Division of Plenum Publishing Corporation
233 Spring Street, New York, N. Y. 10013

10 9 8 7 6 5 4 3 2 1

In memory of my mother,
Bertha Bickman, a woman who
loved children

—LB

Foreword

I am very pleased to see the publication of a book describing the evaluation of the Fort Bragg Child and Adolescent Mental Health Demonstration Project. Earlier presentations and publications addressed parts of the evaluation of this very comprehensive system of services. This book provides an organized compilation of the information from the conceptualization stage through the analysis and interpretation of the first 18 months of data. The description of the evaluation process provides guidance for the design of future studies and the findings reported offer a foundation on which to build future studies of program implementation, quality, costs, and outcomes.

The demonstration project represents the first major effort to execute a fully funded, comprehensive system of care for children and adolescents with a full range of mental health and substance abuse problems and for their families. As such, the evaluation of the system of care is an important contribution to the fields of mental health services and mental health services evaluation. Although both the service system and the evaluation of the system were well designed and comprehensive, they are not without flaws. It is the task of future work to identify the flaws and to make improvements in the design, execution, and interpretation of both the service system and its evaluation.

As the director of the demonstration project and the person with overall responsibility for both the provision of services to the children and adolescents and their families and for the evaluation of the service system, I am proud of the product. The team handling the service system and the team handling the evaluation, by necessity, functioned independently. One of my tasks was to ensure that the points at which their work intersected went smoothly. It has been a pleasure to work with such highly skilled and wonderfully responsive professionals, who always showed respect for each other and had the best interests of the children, adolescents, and their families at heart.

LENORE B. BEHAR

Head, Child and Family Services Branch
North Carolina Division of Mental Health,
*   Developmental Disabilities, and Substance Abuse Services*
Raleigh, North Carolina

Preface

Managed care is often promoted as a means of controlling costs while maintaining the quality of mental health care. Almost half of all Americans are in some form of a managed behavioral health plan. However, the mental health field has been late to recognize the importance of this transformation of service delivery. No controlled studies report on the cost, quality, and mental health outcomes of any of the varieties of managed care in mental health.

Fueled by concerns about escalating expenditures for mental health services and about quality of care, Congress and the Department of Defense have funded several demonstrations of various methods of managing service delivery. The Fort Bragg Evaluation is the first study to examine the provision of a full continuum of mental health services to children and adolescents with mental health and substance abuse problems. This book describes the complex study of this $80 million demonstration funded by the Army and by the National Institute of Mental Health.

Developed under the leadership of Dr. Lenore Behar, a pioneer in the child and adolescent mental health field, the Demonstration provided a full range of mental health services tailored to the needs of children with mental health and substance abuse problems and their families. The continuum of care included residential, intermediate, and nonresidential services with case managers and interdisciplinary treatment teams to integrate treatment programs, facilitate transition between services, and ensure that children were treated in the least restrictive environment.

The American Psychological Association has identified the Demonstration as the most comprehensive program of children's services to date, with available services adaptable to meet the needs of children and their families. The Demonstration was recognized for its provision of a continuum of care in a single location and for its close ties to other services and agencies.

Strong national support exists for the continuum-of-care model and similar concepts, such as systems of care or integrated services. It is common sense to advocate for a system that is based on reducing unnecessary duplication, managing scarce resources, serving children in a less restrictive environment, and generally making it easier for a family to receive needed services. However, it was critical to examine if these notions could be implemented in actual field settings to produce the effects that were generally expected. The Fort Bragg Evaluation was designed to determine whether or not a continuum of services would result in improved treatment outcomes while reducing treatment costs. The Demonstration has provided a rare opportunity to examine both costs and clinical outcomes over time in a thorough evaluation of the implementation of an innovative system of care.

The Evaluation, conducted by the Center for Mental Health Policy at Vanderbilt University, consisted of four substudies: the Implementation Study, the Quality Study, the Mental Health Outcome Study, and the Cost/ Utilization Study. The Implementation and Quality studies focused on documenting the Demonstration's activities. They were designed to assess the degree to which the Demonstration implemented a high-quality system of care that was faithful to the program model. The Mental Health Outcome Study collected data from a sample of children and their families to determine the impact of the Demonstration on child and adolescent psychopathology and psychosocial functioning. The Cost/Utilization Study compared the actual use and cost of services for all treated children. This book focuses primarily on the latter two studies.

The results of this study are surprising. Fundamental current beliefs are challenged. The findings raise critical questions about the effectiveness of mental health services and their delivery in community settings. The results underscore our belief that the way to provide better services is to incorporate scientific program evaluation into program development and system reform efforts.

LEONARD BICKMAN
PAMELA R. GUTHRIE
E. MICHAEL FOSTER
E. WARREN LAMBERT
WM. THOMAS SUMMERFELT
CAROLYN S. BREDA
CRAIG ANNE HEFLINGER

Nashville, Tennessee

Acknowledgments

The Project reported in this book owes its existence to Dr. Lenore Behar. It was her vision in 1986 that brought together a small group to plan the Demonstration and Evaluation Project. It was her persistence and grit that got the Demonstration funded in the face of many roadblocks. Her intellectual integrity has helped maintain the independence of the Evaluation Project. Finally, her desire to know what truly improves the lives of children has helped in the interpretation and dissemination of the findings. Dr. Behar has been assisted, as has the Evaluation Project, by her very able Project Manager, Ed Brannock.

We would also like to thank the many hundreds of children and their families for their cooperation. Without their help, there would have been no Outcome Study. Because of these families, this report will provide guidance in seeking more effective ways to serve children and families.

The staff members at Health Services Command were helpful in securing and interpreting CHAMPUS cost and utilization data. Dr. Scott Optenberg, especially, assisted the Project in numerous ways.

The Rumbaugh Clinic staff and management were of great assistance in the conducting of the Project. They provided data, and assistance in the interpretation of these data, throughout the Project's life. In particular, Dr. Ted Lane and Dr. Pres Keeton helped ensure that our interpretation of the data made sense.

Service providers in the Fort Campbell and Fort Stewart catchment areas provided vital support to the participant recruitment process. Providers at all sites, as well as teachers and school superintendents, were also highly cooperative in providing data.

A number of consultants assisted us throughout this project. An advisory committee met and reflected on our plans, helping to ensure that the Evaluation Project was realistic and answered important questions. We would like to thank: Robert O. Begtrup, Barbara Burns, Mary Jane England, Robert Friedman, Kay Hodges, Kelly Kelleher, Charles A. Kiesler, Thomas McGuire, Leonard Saxe, and Richard Surles.

When preliminary findings were available, we asked a panel of experts to come to Vanderbilt, discuss the findings, and suggest alternative analytical strategies. This panel was very helpful at a critical stage of the Project. We are grateful to: Adrian Angold, Lenore Behar, Ed Brannock, Richard Frank, Robert Friedman, Howard Goldman, Kimberly Hoagwood, Phil Leaf, and Fred Newman.

When a draft of this report was completed, we asked another group of experts to provide feedback on the report within a week. This group provided excellent feedback and helped shape the final document. Our thanks go to: Lenore Behar, Ed Brannock, Gary DeCarolis, Kimberly Hoagwood, Kay Hodges, Ben Lahey, John Landsverk, Ted Lane, Barry Nurcombe, and Bahr Weiss.

Clinical interviews for the Outcome Study were conducted by: Kay Bennet, Lorraine Bonito, Charles Brown, Melba Conley, Jackie Cook, Thomas (Chris) Dempster, Michelle Duffy, Hollie Farris, Lisa Frampton, Dolores Fowler, Brenda Garrett, Tammie Gwiazdowski, Clair Hodge, Cindy Jacobson, Denise James, Jo MacMillan, Gloria Morrow, Kristine Rice, Marvin Roberson, Dale Roussin, Rosemary Scott, Lamar Tillman, Luvi Valino, Daniel Ward, Catherine Warth, David Williams, and Debra Wolraich. In addition, some persons who began working with the Evaluation as interviewers accepted positions on the Vanderbilt staff shortly after, or even before, interviewer training. Interviewer training and monitoring were provided by Sarah Ring-Kurtz and Tonia Hardyway.

Vanderbilt staff worked long and hard to complete this project. Over 5 years, at Fort Bragg, the staff included: Denise Breheny, Sheryl Brewer, Janice Farringer, Katherine Grasso, Charles Grubb, Barbara Harter, Eartha Jacobs, Denise James, Kimberly Pirilla, Mary Ramsey, and Christine Wellborn.

At Fort Campbell: Lisa Grupe, Susan Hewitt, and Olivia Underwood.

At Fort Stewart: Charles Gordon, George Martin, Jr., and Elizabeth Unterseher.

At Vanderbilt: Rebecca Ackley, Bonita Armstrong, MeLissa Benell, Ryan Bennett, Joshua Berger, Corinne Bickman, Felicia Blackmon, Jeanie Boyd, Ana Maria Brannan, Deborah Bryant, Catherine Burciaga, Rebecca Claytor, Julie Conn, Jerome Cook, Kenneth Davis, Vivian Dixon, Robbie Douglas, Susan Douglas, Elizabeth Earl, Dianne Eberhard, Gwen Elferdink, Mark Evans, Jennie Firth, Frederick Bryce Freeman, George Gabriel, Karl Hamner, Tonia Hardyway, Terrell Hayes, Brian Heston, Catherine

Hicks, Petrina Jones, Marc Karver, Jennifer Kinsella, Luann Klindworth, John Kurtz, Shin-Jong (Joy) Lin, Mark Lipsey, Wendi Lozada-Smith, Erin Maloney, Kathleen Maloy, Ann Marable, Jules Marquart, Jan Marra, Suzanne McMurphy, Mary Miles, Donna Miller, Heung Sung Nito, Carol Nixon, Robert Noell, Denine Northrup, Barry Nurcombe, Pamela Pappas, Heather Perry, Keith Peterson, Georgine Pion, Lewis Pollak, Mark Powell, Katherine Price, Dee Rajan, Kristen Raney, Sarah Ring-Kurtz, Debra Rog, Cliff Russell, Howard Sandler, Robert Saunders, James Schut, Tonya Simmons, Celeste (Geri) Simpkins, Michele Sokoly, Carol Solomon, Susan Sonnichsen, Theresa Sparks, Jill Stewart, Zvi Strassberg, Anne Marie Talbott, John Tichenor, John Tongate, Kimberly Vaden, Dee Warmath, Timothy Whang, Barbara White, Jennifer Williams, J. Wilson, and Sam Worley.

Vanderbilt staff members who deserve special recognition are: Craig Anne Heflinger, Jules Marquart, Ana Maria Brannan, and Pamela Guthrie, who served as Project Managers. Carolyn Breda served as Data Manager. Dianne Eberhard provided expertise without which the administrative needs of the Project could never have been met. Denise Breheny, Janice Farringer, Charles Grubb, Lisa Grupe, Susan Hewitt, George Martin, Jr., Kimberly Pirilla, Wendi Lozada-Smith, Olivia Underwood, and Christine Welborn served as Site Coordinators. Finally, staff who devoted themselves to the timely completion and production of this book were Donna Miller, Anne Marie Talbott, MeLissa Benell, and Jennie Firth.

To all these extraordinary people, our heartfelt thanks: Leonard Bickman, Pamela R. Guthrie, E. Michael Foster, E. Warren Lambert, W. Thomas Summerfelt, Carolyn S. Breda, and Craig Anne Heflinger.

This research is supported by the United States Army Health Services Command (DADA 10-89-C-0013) as a subcontract from the North Carolina Department of Human Resources, Division of Mental Health, Developmental Disabilities and Substance Abuse Services, and a grant to Dr. Leonard Bickman (R01MH-46136-01) from the National Institute of Mental Health.

Contents

Tables and Figures

Tables

Figures

1

Introduction

CHILDREN'S MENTAL HEALTH SERVICE SYSTEM ISSUES

The manner in which mental health services are typically provided to children[1] is problematic. Many children receive inappropriate services or no services at all. In the past two decades, many experts (e.g., Cohen, Singh, Hosick, & Tremaine, 1992; Hobbs, 1982; Knitzer, 1982; Stroul & Friedman, 1986) have highlighted the vast discrepancy between the numbers of children in need of mental health services and those who receive appropriate services. It is estimated that 11–20% of all children are in need of mental health services (Brandenburg, Friedman, & Silver, 1990; Costello, 1989; Saxe, Cross, & Silverman, 1988). More than half these children receive no treatment, and many who are treated receive inappropriate care (Davis, Yelton, & Katz-Leavy, 1993; Knitzer, 1993; Saxe et al., 1988). An estimated 80% of children needing services receive inappropriate care or none at all (Inouye, 1988).

There is also agreement that unnecessarily restrictive treatment settings are overutilized (Dorwart, Schelsinger, Davidson, Epstein, & Hoover, 1991; National Mental Health Association, 1989; Weithorn, 1988). It is believed that children with emotional problems are best treated in the least restrictive, most normative environment that is clinically feasible (Stroul & Friedman, 1986). However, the number of private psychiatric hospitals showed continued growth during the 1980s (Bickman & Dokecki, 1989; Frank & Dewa, 1992) due to the tendency to finance mental health services through the hospital-based medical model (Kiesler, 1992). Reimbursement

[1]We recognize that the terms "children," "adolescents," "teenagers," "youth," and others are not always perfectly interchangeable. However, to avoid confusion and for consistency, the term "children" will be used throughout this book to refer to persons in all these age groups.

incentives have encouraged use of the most restrictive levels of care, in lieu of less restrictive community-based services. The best estimate to date (Burns, 1991) is that more than 75% of the funding for children's mental health services nationwide is spent on institutional care. The use of residential mental health treatment is much greater than even those figures suggest, once one considers a broader system perspective that includes general hospitals (Kiesler & Simpkins, 1991, 1993).

Contributing to the problem of unnecessarily restrictive treatment is the general unavailability of alternative treatment settings (Knitzer, 1993). Knitzer (1982), Behar (1985), and Silver (1984) estimated that 40% of inpatient placements were inappropriate, either because the children could have been treated in less restrictive settings or because initially appropriate placements were no longer appropriate and less restrictive treatment settings were not available. In a follow-up survey of state mental health administrators, Davis et al. (1993) found that several problems identified by Knitzer (1982) had been addressed in some ways. However, inappropriate placements continue, such as out-of-state residential placements and treatment of children in adult psychiatric hospital units. These practices contradict widely held beliefs that even children with severe emotional disturbances (SED) can receive treatment while living in their own homes, if a comprehensive system of care is present in the community (Behar, 1985).

Even where services are available, it is believed that the lack of coordination between them compromises the effectiveness of the interventions (Cohen et al., 1992; Fagan, 1991; Saxe, Cross, Silverman, Batchelor, & Dougherty, 1987; Schmitz & Gilchrist, 1991; Soler & Shauffer, 1990; Stroul & Friedman, 1986). Given the developmental complexity and multiple needs of children, it is strongly believed that services should be both available and coordinated if they are to address the needs of these children effectively (Behar, 1985; Rog, 1992).

The concept of integrated, comprehensive systems of care for children was developed in response to problems concerning the availability and delivery of mental health services for children (Stroul & Friedman, 1986). In their seminal work, Stroul and Friedman outlined the guiding principles and components critical to an accessible, comprehensive, appropriate, and cost-effective system of care for children. The term system of care encompasses this philosophy of treatment and the organizational structures and mechanisms necessary for the implementation of a truly coordinated, multiagency service-delivery system (Stroul, 1994). A cornerstone of such a system of care is the availability of a full range of mental health services designed to meet most appropriately the varied and changing needs of children with emotional and behavioral disorders and their families.

This array of treatments has been termed a continuum of care (Stroul & Friedman, 1986) and includes residential, intermediate, and nonresidential services. The emphasis on intermediate-level services that has emerged includes attempts to deliver needed services on an individualized basis and in a coordinated manner, relying on case management and interdisciplinary treatment teams to integrate treatment programs and facilitate transition between services. The continuum is also designed to be community-based, involving various agencies pertinent to children's developmental, educational, medical, and mental health needs.

While there has been noteworthy progress (Davis et al., 1993; Friedman & Kutash, 1992; Knitzer, 1993) in the years since the publication of the Stroul and Friedman (1986) guidelines, experts in the field maintain that such services continue to be underfunded, lacking interagency coordination and sufficient research-generated knowledge base to support the appropriateness, effectiveness, and cost-efficiency of different mental health services for children with emotional and behavioral disorders (Burchard & Schaefer, 1992; Cohen et al., 1992; Friedman & Kutash, 1992; Knitzer, 1993; Oswald, Singh, & Ellis, 1992; Schmitz & Gilchrist, 1991; VandenBos, 1993).

There are many other impediments to the development of reliable and useful evaluative research in the area of children's mental health services (Rog, 1992). Limited funding of such services has resulted in very few opportunities to evaluate empirically the effectiveness of the system-of-care or continuum-of-care approach (Davis et al., 1993; Friedman & Kutash, 1992; Schmitz & Gilchrist, 1991). Studies typically lack random assignment of service recipients or adequate comparison groups or are subject to the complexities inherent in longitudinal research (Burchard & Schaefer, 1992; Rig, 1992). In addition to other challenges, researchers in this field have had to rely on a limited knowledge base in their efforts to study these complex systems of service delivery. Very little is known about systems of care and how to study them (Burns, 1994).

The field of children's mental health service delivery is additionally facing challenges related to the recent debate about health care reform in the United States. Health care reform is being developed, debated, and scrutinized and will influence and be influenced by mental health research (VandenBos, 1993). Advocates of the coordinated system of care stress the importance of maintaining the growing paradigmatic shift away from institution-based treatment to ensure funding of less restrictive community-based services (Knitzer, 1993). Both Kiesler (1992) and VandenBos (1993) agree that current financing structures rely inappropriately on a hospital-based health policy framework, thus perpetuating the increase in and continued use of residential facilities to treat children. Frank and Dewa

(1992) point out that while use of inpatient services has increased, demand for outpatient mental health services has grown at a faster rate, and there has been no empirical evidence to challenge the appropriateness of the existing distribution of available services. Many authors assert that mental health policy should not be treated simply as an extension of health policy (Friedman & Kutash, 1992; Kiesler, 1992; VandenBos, 1993). However, efforts to view it differently will require radical changes in the current financing and incentive structure for all mental health services. With cost containment a top priority in health policy, mental health benefits may be constrained to a "cost-effective minimum benefit package" (Durenberger & Foote, 1993). However, the determination of interventions and services that are cost-effective depends solely on the availability and quality of services research and evaluation information, which is still limited (Knitzer, 1993; Oswald et al., 1992; Rog, 1992; Bickman & Rog, 1995).

Changes in innovative financing structures have not yet been linked to treatment effectiveness (Durenberger & Foote, 1993; Friedman & Kutash, 1992; Oswald et al., 1992; VandenBos, 1993), but efforts are currently under way to address challenges in providing children's mental health services. Concerns about large expenditures for mental health services and quality of care, especially for children and adolescents, have motivated the Congress and the Department of Defense to fund and implement a number of demonstrations of different service delivery mechanisms. These managed care[2] experiments share two major goals: to control costs and to maintain or enhance quality of services. The Fort Bragg Demonstration and Evaluation Projects were the first and largest attempts to study an innovative approach to service delivery for children and adolescents with mental health problems. The Fort Bragg Child and Adolescent Mental Health Demonstration (hereinafter referred to as the Demonstration) and the Fort Bragg Evaluation Project (Project) were designed to:

- Test the "efficacy of a Federal and State contract for providing a case management–based alternative delivery system of mental health services tailored to individual needs featuring the use of a full continuum of community-based services."
- "Demonstrate that this continuum of services [would] result in

---

[2]"The term 'managed care,' lacking a commonly accepted definition, has been used to characterize a wide range of health care plans. Some employers broadly define managed care to include all plans that incorporate mechanisms to monitor and authorize the use of health services. Others more narrowly define managed care to include only health plans that direct enrollees to selected physicians and hospitals with which the plan has negotiated payment methods and utilization controls" (General Accounting Office, 1993c).

improved treatment outcomes while the cost of care per client is decreased when compared to current CHAMPUS costs."[3]

In addition to the Fort Bragg Demonstration, two other demonstrations and the passage of federal legislation are relevant to the study of systems of care in mental health. Two major demonstration projects, sponsored by the Robert Wood Johnson Foundation (RWJF), have been conducted concurrently with the Demonstration. Like the Demonstration, they examined the implementation and effects of integrating mental health services through a centralized system of care. Unlike the Demonstration, they were broader in scope. They attempted to demonstrate how multiple public agencies could pool resources and develop and implement a system of care. The RWJF provided funds for project management, technical assistance, program evaluation, and case management. Communities were then required to develop the financing models needed to support the full array of services necessary to treat clients. In contrast, the Demonstration had a single source of funds for the development and management of the system as well as for all services.

The RWJF Program on Chronic Mental Illness was initiated in 1986 with funding of $29 million for 5 years. In this program, 9 of the 60 largest United States cities participated to help adults with chronic mental illness function better in their everyday lives. The program model specified that a centralized mental health authority would result in expanded services and resources and thus improve client outcomes. The summative evaluation was funded by the National Institute of Mental Health and the RWJF. The evaluators concluded that "... a mental authority might be necessary, but not sufficient to create a comprehensive system of services. Most of the cities improved the availability of services, especially case management, but none had a truly comprehensive system of community support services by the end of the demonstration" (Goldman, Morrissey, & Ridgely, 1994, p. 42). Thus, it is not surprising that the evaluators found that this demonstration had no significant effect on client outcomes, such as quality of life, when compared with other sites. In general, the evaluators concluded that case management and structural changes were not sufficient to bring about change at the individual client level. They felt that without the addition of appropriate services, there should be no expectation that

---

[3]Contract DADA 10-89-R-0013 between the Army Health Services Command and the North Carolina Department of Human Resources, Division of Mental Health, Developmental Disabilities, and Substance Abuse Services, p. C-1, Amendment 0001. CHAMPUS refers to the insurer of dependent, the Civilian Health and Medical Program of the Uniformed Services.

clients' lives would change (Goldman et al., 1994; Lehman, Postrado, Roth, McNary, & Goldman, 1994; Shern, Wilson, & Coen, 1994).

The Mental Health Services Program for Youth (MHSPY) was similar to the adult demonstration. In 1989, 8 states were funded for 5 years for $20.4 million to integrate the service systems for children with serious emotional disturbances. Again, this program differed from the Demonstration model in that the interaction of several public systems of care was required, and new funds for direct services were not provided by the foundation. It was similar to the Demonstration in its focus on children and was based on continuum-of-care principles that supported a full array of services (Cole & Poe, 1993). The results of the program evaluation of the MHSPY, conducted by Brandeis University, will not be available until late 1995. However, the evaluation did not include collection of comprehensive and systematic outcome data at the client level. Further, it did not include a Comparison site and apparently assumed that if the service system changed, then client outcomes would also change. Thus, the data collection and the design of the evaluation will not allow causal inferences about the effect of the demonstration on clinical outcomes.

A major milestone in children's mental health services was the passage of the Comprehensive Community Mental Health Services Program for Children and Adolescents with Severe Emotional Disturbances (SED), signed into law on July 10, 1992 (Part E of Title V, section 561 *et seq.* of the Public Health Service Act). The program, which was originally authorized for funding at over $100 million per year, and in 1994 actually distributed over $35 million, encompasses systems of care in 38 different localities. The grant provides funds for assessment, case management, outpatient treatment, day treatment, in-home services, respite care, therapeutic foster care, and group homes for children with SED. These services are the basis of a continuum of care, central to the grant program. The federally funded evaluation that is planned for this program is not designed, however, to determine whether the continuum of care results in changes in clinical outcomes. Clearly, the Demonstration and this program share a common heritage and are based on similar principles. The results of this Project are very relevant to this major federal grant program.

The Department of Defense (DOD) has funded a number of demonstration projects, primarily to reduce costs of the Civilian Health and Medical Program of the Uniformed Services (CHAMPUS). Baine (1992) reported that these managed care projects in Hawaii, California, and Tidewater, Virginia, all demonstrated that utilization review procedures can reduce costs by reducing admissions and length of stay in inpatient facilities. However, he noted that because the contractors in these sites had fixed contract prices that put them at financial risk, there have been significant questions raised about the "... efficacy of their utilization review activities. A recent congressional hearing in the Tidewater area focused on these concerns. Also, RAND data raise some concerns in California and Hawaii, because of high inpatient readmission rates in the two states" (Baine, 1992, p. 189). None of these demonstrations assessed the clinical outcomes of care, so it is not possible to determine whether their utilization review activities negatively affected clinical outcomes.

The evaluation of the Demonstration has provided a rare opportunity to examine costs and clinical outcomes over time. Further, it has provided an opportunity to examine the continuum-of-care concept in the context of a thorough evaluation of the implementation of both the innovative and standard systems of care (see Heflinger, 1993).

THE FORT BRAGG DEMONSTRATION
AND EVALUATION PROJECTS

The Demonstration was based on the continuum-of-care philosophy. Before describing in greater detail the Demonstration and its evaluation, however, we first discuss the typical services that are provided to dependents insured under CHAMPUS.

Traditional CHAMPUS Services

Benefits

In fiscal year 1991, CHAMPUS changed its benefit structure to allow 45 days of inpatient or hospital care, 150 days of residential treatment center (RTC) care, and 23 outpatient visits per year. These changes reflected a reduction in coverage for outpatient and inpatient days and the imposition of a limit for RTC days. It should be noted that most private insurance does not cover care in an RTC. CHAMPUS also covers about twice the number of outpatient visits that many private insurers cover. Under CHAMPUS, no lifetime benefit or dollar limit is imposed, as is the case with many other insurers (Baine, 1992). CHAMPUS requires a $150 deductible per person and $300 per family per year for all families except those of active-duty E-4 and below. Family members of active-duty E-4 and below pay $50 per person and $100 for the family. A copayment of 20% of allowable charges is paid by active-duty families and 25% of allowable charges is paid by all other families (OCHAMPUS, 1992).[4] CHAMPUS also

---

[4]A copayment of 15% is required when seeing a CHAMPUS-Select provider.

provides for a "catastrophic cap" on out-of-pocket expenditures on allowable charges of $1000 for active-duty dependents and $7500 for others.[5] For families with other health insurance in addition to CHAMPUS benefits, CHAMPUS pays only after all other plans' benefits have been exhausted, except for Medicaid and certain insurance policies that are specifically designate as CHAMPUS supplements.

Cost Reduction

The high cost of providing mental health services to the children of military personnel motivated CHAMPUS to consider alternatives to the existing delivery system and to implement a variety of demonstration programs. In 1983, CHAMPUS alone spent $74 million on inpatient mental health hospitalization for dependent children. Between 1985 and 1989, mental health care costs for children and adults doubled to more than $600 million per year, although the number of beneficiaries remained relatively constant. Inpatient care increased from $200 million to almost $500 million in the same 5-year period (1985–1989), and mental health care to children in hospitals and RTCs accounted for 3 of every 4 days of total inpatient mental health care. Between 1989 and 1991, CHAMPUS mental health costs stabilized. In 1991, costs totaled approximately $631 million, with inpatient costs accounting for 79%, or $500 million. Moreover, about $305 million was spent for treatment of children, with approximately $164 million being paid to RTCs (Baine, 1992).

Effective (on a voluntary basis) since January 1, 1990, and made mandatory on October 1, 1991, Health Management Strategies International, Inc., (HMS) was responsible for providing utilization management for all inpatient and residential treatment facility stays and for outpatient visits exceeding 23 visits per annum for CHAMPUS-covered care. The DOD judged that "because the main area of runaway costs and skyrocketing utilization and LOS [length of stay] involved residential care of adolescents, the Department concentrated a great deal of attention on this type of care. This was accomplished through a contract with HMS for utilization management" (Martin, 1992, p. 219). From 1990 to 1991, the DOD reported a decrease in LOS for both hospitalization and RTCs.

While total CHAMPUS costs increased in fiscal year 1991, mental health costs declined slightly (0.26%). Between 1990 and 1991, average LOS

[5]During the course of the Demonstration, the cap was lowered to $7500 from $10,000. The cap is important because when out-of-pocket expenses exceed the cap, cost-sharing no longer applies. From a consumer's perspective, services are free. At the Demonstration site, services are provided without charge (so that, effectively, there is no cap).

in RTCs dropped from 188 days to 136 days and in acute hospitalization from 23.6 days to 18.6 days. While LOS decreased, RTC costs continued to increase. The number of RTC admissions went up 13%, and admission for inpatient substance abuse rose 65% during this period (Martin, 1992). The number of hospital admissions also increased 17%.

As part of the comprehensive effort to reduce the high CHAMPUS costs associated with the delivery of health care and mental health care to military families, a program of coordinated care involving more stringent preauthorization requirements, some treatment restrictions, and a revised schedule of deductibles and copayments was implemented effective April 1, 1991 (October 1, 1991, for Persian Gulf participants). The program was administered by Health Management Strategies International, Inc., the CHAMPUS mental health utilization review contractor. These limits were subject to special waiver or limited extension, however, if medical necessity could be demonstrated to the mental health contractor.

One coordinated care effort made local hospital commanders responsible for managing expenditures in their catchment areas. Under this Gateway to Care Program (Gateway), more beneficiaries are treated in military hospitals in an attempt to decrease purchase of services through CHAMPUS. Gateway's impact on the Project is discussed in Chapter 5.

Significant controversy exists about the efficacy of managed care systems. The application of a variety of managed care schemes to children's mental health services by CHAMPUS has recently been discussed in a congressional hearing (Select Committee, 1992). Furthermore, studies dealing with some CHAMPUS reform initiatives are themselves surrounded by controversy (General Accounting Office, 1992, 1993a,b); these previous evaluations dealt only with cost and utilization. The Project is the first comprehensive evaluation of a continuum of care, provided within a system that utilizes managed care components, and includes the assessment of mental health outcomes.

The Fort Bragg Demonstration Project

In 1986, Dr. Lenore Behar, Director of Children's Services for the North Carolina Department of Human Resources, Division of Mental Health, Developmental Disabilities, and Substance Abuse Services (DMH/DD/SAS), and a nationally known consultant on children's mental health services, developed the Demonstration concept. By 1987, she had convened a small group to plan a program and an evaluation of a system of care that would be an alternative to traditional CHAMPUS services. After much negotiation and many setbacks in planning between the State of North Carolina (State) and the DOD, Congress requested the Department of the Army (Army), in August 1989, to fund the Demonstration and an independent evaluation (the Project) through a contract with the DMH/DD/SAS.

The DMH/DD/SAS contracted with Cardinal Mental Health Group, Inc. (Cardinal), a private, not-for-profit corporation located in Fayetteville, North Carolina, to provide a continuum of care for the Fort Bragg catchment area, an approximate 40-mile radius surrounding the Army post. The funding for the subcontract to Cardinal was directed through a local government agency, the Lee-Harnett Area MH/DD/SAS program. Cardinal's contract restricted its services to eligible military dependents under the age of 18. On June 1, 1990, after a 10-month start-up period, mental health and substance abuse services were offered to a population that included over 42,000 child dependents of military personnel in the Fort Bragg area. The initial subcontract established a 4-year period for the Demonstration. However, the services contract between the Army and the State has been extended through September 1995.

Using a closed system or exclusive provider organization model, the Demonstration required that families seeking services for their children either use the Demonstration's clinical services (which required no copayment or deductible and thus were free) or seek and pay for services on their own. The range of services included both community-based nonresidential and residential treatment components.[6] Cardinal contracted with individuals and agencies in the community already providing traditional mental health services, such as outpatient therapy and acute inpatient hospitalization, and itself provided intensive outpatient treatment. For the middle or intermediate level of the continuum (those services neither previously available in Fayetteville nor typically available across the country), Cardinal developed services that included in-home therapy, after-school group treatment, day treatment, therapeutic homes, specialized group homes, and 24-hour crisis management teams. All children requesting services were to receive a comprehensive intake and assessment to determine the appropriate level of care. Cardinal services were provided through the Major General James H. Rumbaugh, Jr., Child and Adolescent Mental Health Clinic (Rumbaugh Clinic).[7]

---

[6]See Chapter 4 and Chapter 5 for descriptions of the intake/assessment and treatment components of the Demonstration.

[7]Cardinal holds the contract to provide services for the Demonstration through the Rumbaugh Clinic. These entities/agencies are not synonymous. Throughout this book, "Demonstration" is used as a general term to avoid confusion. However, in some instances, the authors felt that this general convention did not clearly identify the subject of the discussion. In these cases, the term "Cardinal" or "the Rumbaugh Clinic" has been used to denote that agency as the focus of discussion.

For children using intermediate or more intensive-level services, the clinical services were to be coordinated with the other child-serving agencies and practitioners in the community, especially pediatric, educational, and protective services. Services within the continuum and across other agencies were linked through a case management component and interdisciplinary treatment teams led by a doctoral-level staff person. Data regarding these services are provided in Chapter 5. Related services, such as transportation and other wraparound services, designed to provide individualized support in any setting, were also provided. More detailed descriptions of the services can be found in the final report of the implementation study (Heflinger, 1993) and in Behar, Bickman, Lane, Keeton, and Schwartz (1995).

The Demonstration has been recognized as providing model services to children. The American Psychological Association's section on Child Clinical Psychology and the Division of Child, Youth and Family Services formed a task force to identify, recognize, and disseminate information on interventions that best meet child and family needs (Roberts, 1994). The Demonstration was considered a model program because it was seen as "... the most comprehensive program to date, integrating many of the approaches demonstrated by other service programs" and its approach was considered "... integrated and flexibly constructed, yet comprehensive, [with] services ... available to be adapted to meet the needs of children and their families, rather than a simplistic application of a single approach to all presenting problems" (Roberts, 1994, p. 215). The Demonstration was also lauded for its provision of a continuum of care in a single location and its close ties to other services and agencies.

The Demonstration required no financial outlay for the families. The usual copayments and deductibles were waived. The assumption was that since the families had no practical choice but to utilize the Demonstration if they needed services, they should receive some compensation for their loss of choice of providers. Moreover, the waiving of the deductible eliminated some difficult accounting problems for the Army. A cost-reimbursement contract allowed the Demonstration to best initiate a continuum of care. Little was known about how many children previously unserved might enter the system or about exactly what services would be needed. Rather than place any restriction on services based solely on financial issues, the Army preferred to reimburse the Demonstration for services it actually provided. Since this project was initiated as a cost-reimbursement contract, theoretically no limits were placed on the types or costs of services to be offered as long as they were therapeutically appropriate. The Demonstration was to provide the best possible services for children without the usual limitations placed on providers by insurance companies or other public agencies. Thus, the Demonstration was to be a test of the continuum-of-care model without the usual financial constraints or implementation problems found when multiple agencies are required to collaborate and pool funds.

The philosophy of the Demonstration called for controlling costs, not by the conventional mode of placing a limit or cap on services or cost per child, but by providing a continuum of services designed to be more appropriate for each child. Since there was little or no financial incentive for the Demonstration to provide inappropriate services, it was hypothesized that this rational/clinical approach to managing benefits would be a more effective means of controlling costs than placing fixed limits on care. However, lack of cost-sharing by parents may have removed one mechanism to limit unnecessary services; research has documented that use of mental health services by children is influenced by the extent to which their parents share the costs of those services (Padgett, Patrick, Burns, Schlesinger, & Cohen, 1992; Patrick, Padgett, Burns, Schlesinger, & Cohen, 1993; Tsai, Reedy, Bernacki, & Lee, 1988). Given this influence, however, the Demonstration did operate under the scrutiny of the State, the Army, and Congress, and was under some pressure to provide the most cost-effective treatment possible (see Chapter 7).

The Fort Bragg Evaluation Project

The Center for Mental Health Policy of the Vanderbilt Institute for Public Policy Studies at Vanderbilt University was awarded a subcontract by the DMH/DD/SAS to conduct an independent evaluation of the Demonstration. The Evaluation Project consisted of four substudies: (1) Implementation Study, (2) Quality Study, (3) Mental Health Outcome Study, and (4) Cost/Utilization Study.

The Implementation and Quality Studies were devoted to documenting the Demonstration's activities. The primary purpose of these two substudies was to assess the degree to which the Demonstration implemented a high-quality system of care and was faithful to the program model that is discussed below. The final reports of the implementation and quality studies were completed in September 1993. These documents are cited throughout this book where relevant. To summarize their results briefly:

- The Implementation Study (Heflinger, 1993) provided a comprehensive description of how the Demonstration was put in place. It presented evidence necessary to conclude that the Demonstration was executed with sufficient fidelity, despite barriers, to provide an

excellent test of the continuum of care and to meaningfully examine program outcomes and costs.
- The Quality Study (Bickman, Bryant, & Summerfelt, 1993) provided evidence that key components of service were of sufficient quality to produce the theoretically expected positive outcomes.

The Mental Health Outcome Study, one of the two substudies reported here, was quasi-experimental and longitudinal. A sample of children and their families at the Demonstration site and at the Comparison site provided data to determine the relative impact of the Demonstration on the psychopathology and psychosocial functioning of children, as well as on family well-being. Initial (baseline) mental health outcome data were collected within approximately 30 days after entry into the service system, followed by two additional outcome data collection waves approximately 6 months apart. Extensive and complex recruitment procedures, described more fully in Chapter 2, were followed to maximize participation in the Evaluation. Because the Evaluation Sample was weighted toward those receiving the most intensive care, and since participation was voluntary, the sample participating was not representative of the total population treated. However, information presented in Chapter 3 examines similarities and differences between the Evaluation Sample and others receiving treatment in diagnostic, service utilization, and demographic characteristics.

It is important to note that in all discussions of participant samples in the following chapters, three groups are distinguished in the Project. The Evaluation Sample was composed of the 984 children and their families who participated in the Mental Health Outcome Study. However, for some analyses, especially in the Cost-Utilization Study, we were interested in all the children eligible for services within the Project catchment areas. This larger group of children and families is referred to throughout this book as the *catchment population*. Finally, when analyses utilized the subgroup of the catchment population that actually received mental health services, that group is referred to as the *treated population*.

The Cost/Utilization Study compared the actual use of services with the costs of those services for all children treated (including, but not limited to, those participating in the Mental Health Outcome Study) at both the Demonstration site and the Comparison site. The Army selected two comparison sites, Fort Stewart and Fort Campbell, that were similar to the Demonstration site. In almost all discussion that follows, these two sites are referred to jointly as the Comparison site.

Since we were unable to use random assignment of children to different systems of care, the inclusion of a Comparison site was critical to the examination of the effectiveness of the Demonstration (Bickman, 1992).

PROGRAM THEORY

Program theory is "a plausible and sensible model of how a program is supposed to work" (Bickman, 1987, p. 5). Describing the program theory is a critical initial step in evaluation, since hypothesized links between program features and planned outcomes can then be logically tested (Heflinger, 1993).

Several program-evaluation theorists (Bickman, 1987, 1990; Chen & Rossi, 1992; Lipsey, 1990) differentiate between program theory failure and program implementation failure. In the study presented in this book, the theory being tested is that a comprehensive, integrated, and coordinated continuum of care is more cost-effective than a fragmented service system with a limited variety of services. The theory could be tested only if the Demonstration implemented this theory sufficiently well and if our evaluation methods were valid. Since a continuum of care had never before been implemented on this scale, it was not automatically assumed by the Project that such an undertaking would necessarily be successful. Thus, efforts were expended to conceptualize and describe the Demonstration theory and its actual implementation.

Figure 1.1 shows the evaluators' theory of the Demonstration, indicat-

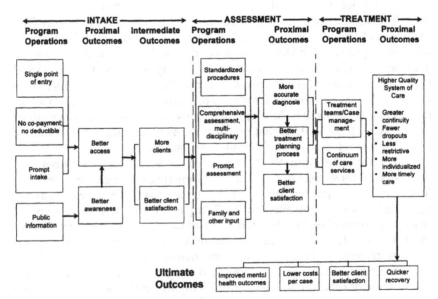

Figure 1.1. Fort Bragg Child and Adolescent Demonstration: Program theory.

ing several underlying assumptions. Most of these assumptions have been tested by the Project. This theory or model serves as the main organizing principle for this book. Chapters 4–8 will focus on aspects of the Demonstration as described in this theoretical model.

At the left side of Figure 1.1 are the intake characteristics of this system. The uppermost box indicates that there is a single point of entry into the system. Unlike many nonsystems or more complex systems, the eligible population can receive mental health services only through the Rumbaugh Clinic, although the clinic may, in turn, utilize contract providers for some services. Families can choose to obtain services outside the system, but they must pay for those services either themselves or through another insurer. This single point of entry is important because it allows the Demonstration to control access to services. Moreover, a single point of entry should make it simple for potential clients to know where mental health services can be obtained. As part of its contract, the Demonstration had to provide services at no cost to the client. Thus, there was no copayment or deductible associated with any service.

Rigorous standards of timeliness are not routinely part of the "services as usual" provided under CHAMPUS. However, as part of its contract with the Army, the DMH/DD/SAS had to ensure that clients would receive intake and subsequent services promptly. The contract originally called for diagnosis and assessment to begin with 1 week after a referral for nonemergency cases, with assessment completed and reviewed by a treatment team within 2 weeks or less. However, because of an unexpectedly high client flow and the obvious expense involved in maintaining this standard and its questionable clinical value, the State convinced the Army that a standard for initiation of assessment within 3 weeks should be set.

As shown in the lower left-hand box of Figure 1.1, at the start of services, the Demonstration was required to engage in a public information or marketing program to inform the providers and potential clients about the new system of care. These activities were hypothesized to produce a *proximal outcome* of increased awareness of and access to services. This increased access should have resulted in two *intermediate outcomes*: (1) an increase in the number of clients served because of the reduced barriers to obtaining services and (2) an increase in client satisfaction with the intake process (over what one would expect from traditional CHAMPUS services) through reduced financial burden and ease of access.

The percentage of the eligible population that received services and the change in this percentage over time are described in Chapter 4, as is client satisfaction.

The middle section of Figure 1.1 illustrates the *program operations* during the *assessment* process. All families were to participate in a standard intake process. This process usually included comprehensive evaluation and a review by an interdisciplinary treatment team. Again, the Demonstration contract set standards for prompt assessment (within 3 weeks), including input from family and other relevant professionals. These program activities were hypothesized to lead to three *proximal outcomes*: (1) a more accurate diagnosis, leading to (2) a better treatment plan and (3) increased client satisfaction with the assessment process.

We expected a more accurate diagnosis because of the comprehensive intake and assessment process, family participation, involvement of the multidisciplinary team, and the fact that reimbursement was not tied to diagnosis. Treatment planning should be improved because of the increased accuracy in judgments of the child's problems. Consumer satisfaction with the assessment process should be improved because of the involvement of the family and the perceived accuracy of the assessment process. These issues are discussed in Chapter 4.

The actual *treatment* (characterized at the right-hand side of Figure 1.1) provided by the Demonstration included management of more complex cases by a treatment team and clinical case manager and access to the wide variety of services available in the continuum of care. As noted earlier, the services offered by the Demonstration included inpatient and residential treatment, in-home therapy, after-school treatment, day treatment, therapeutic homes, specialized group homes, 24-hour crisis management team, wraparound services, and intensive outpatient treatment. These program activities should lead to the *proximal outcome* of a higher-quality system of care that provides a better match between the needs of the child and family and the treatment provided. Operationally defined, a quality system of care:

- Has more continuity between services.
- Has fewer dropouts from treatment.
- Provides services at the most appropriate and least restrictive level of treatment.
- Provides more individualized treatment.
- Has more timely transitions between levels of care.

These activities are discussed in Chapter 5.

The Demonstration should therefore lead to the following *ultimate outcomes* as compared to mental health treatment provided under traditional CHAMPUS: improved mental health, lower costs per case, quicker recovery, and more client satisfaction. The higher-quality service system should increase the probability that treatment will affect the client. While the total costs of the Demonstration may be higher, primarily because of the anticipated increase in the number of clients treated, it is expected that similar cases will cost less to treat at the Demonstration site than at the

Comparison site. However, it is recognized that these last hypotheses may have to be examined together to discern the true effects of the Demonstration. That is, it is expected that for similar cases, the Demonstration will be more cost-effective than traditional care. This ratio of effectiveness to cost is the ultimate outcome considered most important to the Project.

In Chapter 2, the methods employed to collect and manage data for the Project are described. Chapter 3 then describes the Evaluation Sample and its representativeness of populations of interest.

The next four chapters report findings directly related to the program theory outlined above. Mental health outcome, satisfaction with services, utilization of services, and costs are discussed in chapters devoted to the intake and assessment process (Chapter 4), the treatment process (Chapter 5), mental health outcomes (Chapter 6), and cost outcomes (Chapter 7).

Chapter 8 reviews the program theory presented earlier in this chapter and relates this theory to the findings reported in Chapters 4–7. Finally it discusses the policy and implementation implications of our findings.

2

Methods

This chapter reviews the methods by which data were collected and managed for the Mental Health Outcome (Outcome) Study and the Cost/Utilization (C/U) Study. Because the two studies differed in their research questions, they also varied in their methods, including their data collection strategies and samples of interest. It is important to recall that the Outcome Study was based on data collected directly from families recruited for the Evaluation (the Evaluation Sample). The C/U Study was based on data compiled from a variety of secondary sources. Its samples of interest, moreover, included the Evaluation Sample as well as two others—all children in the catchment areas eligible for treatment (catchment population) and all children in the catchment areas who actually received mental health services (treated population).

THE MENTAL HEALTH OUTCOME STUDY

Project Management

The catchment areas for recruitment into the study surrounded Fort Bragg for the Demonstration site and Forts Stewart and Campbell for the Comparison site. Field site offices were established in Fayetteville, North Carolina, Savannah, Georgia, and Nashville, Tennessee, to support recruitment and data collection for each of the respective catchment areas. Site Coordinators supervised operations at each field location and were in turn supervised by the Project Manager, whose office was located in Nashville, Tennessee, on the Vanderbilt University campus. To ensure standardized data collection procedures, a detailed procedures manual was developed and revised over the course of the Project. It served as the primary educational and reference tool for site staff. The Project Manager and other supervisory staff met every other month with all Site Coordinators on the Vanderbilt campus and reviewed data collection procedures and related issues. In addition, the Project Manager or a designated staff member traveled to each site office during the months in which Site Coordinator meetings were not held. During these site visits, record-keeping, data collection techniques, and supervision of field site staff were audited. Thus, although data collection was conducted over a broad geographic area and by many staff members, data were collected similarly at all sites.

Participant Recruitment and Retention

Efforts to recruit participants varied by site. All families at the Demonstration site presented themselves for services through a single point of entry—the Rumbaugh Clinic. Thus, the Clinic referred all prospective study participants to Project staff. Recruitment at the Comparison site was considerably more involved. There, several recruitment strategies were used—most effectively, the establishment of a network of all service providers in the area. Site Coordinators identified service providers through various means, including review of referral lists from Army post Civilian Health and Medical Program of the Uniformed Services (CHAMPUS) offices, community service guides, local phone and professional association directories, and prior CHAMPUS claims. The Coordinators then called the providers, briefly described the Project, and asked them to refer to them new child clients who were using CHAMPUS benefits and had agreed to be contacted by Project staff. Children in inpatient or residential mental health facilities were identified through "Nonavailability of Service" (NAS) forms made available at each post.[1] At all sites, Site Coordinators contacted the prospective participants to establish eligibility and, if a participant was eligible, arrange a face-to-face visit to obtain informed consent.

Children who met the following criteria were eligible to participate:

- Resided in the site's catchment area, defined as about a 40-mile radius from the military post.
- Had a caregiver (e.g., parent) who could act as a reliable informant.

[1]Under CHAMPUS guidelines, a precertification procedure takes place when a child is to enter an inpatient or residential treatment facility. In these cases, a parent must apply for CHAMPUS coverage by specifying that such services are not available through the on-post hospital. The post hospitals do not offer inpatient or residential treatment for children, so an NAS form is filed. These forms were kept on post and were made available for the purpose of identifying children to participate in the Project.

- Were between the ages of 5 and 17.
- Had not been in treatment more than 1 month before Project contact.
- Received services either through Rumbaugh (for Demonstration families) or providers within 75 miles of the post (for Comparison families).
- Were eligible for CHAMPUS benefits.
- Would be living in the area for at least 6 months, until the first follow-up.

The top row of Table 2.1 shows that providers referred more than 2000 families over the 2½ years of recruitment. Most families (93%) were contacted; of them, most (75%) met eligibility criteria. Of eligible families, 61% (N = 984) agreed to participate and completed the initial interview. Recruitment rates varied by site, most notably with regard to the proportion of families eligible and the proportion who completed the interview. However, as will be shown in Chapter 3, there were few clinically related

Table 2.1. Participant Recruitment and Retention

Group	Demonstration N	Demonstration %	Comparison N	Comparison %	Total N	Total %
Referrals	1386	—	947	—	2333	—
Able to contact	1247	90%	916	97%	2163	93%
Eligible	1065	85%	553	60%	1618	75%
Wave 1						
Completed interview	574	54%	410	74%	984	61%
Wave 2	573[b]	—	411[b]	—	984	—
Not located (skipped)[a]	34	6%	20	5%	54	5%
Refused (skipped)[a]	10	2%	6	1%	16	2%
Attrited	6	1%	7	2%	13	1%
Completed						
Without diagnostic data	49	8%	29	7%	78	8%
With diagnostic data	474	83%	349	85%	823	84%
Wave 3						
Not located	67	12%	38	9%	105	11%
Refused	34	6%	21	5%	55	6%
Completed						
Without diagnostic data	71	12%	30	8%	101	10%
With diagnostic data	395	70%	315	78%	710	73%

[a]Cases "skipped" at Wave 2 were followed at Wave 3. Only attrited cases were dropped from the Evaluation.
[b]One family transferred from the Demonstration to a Comparison site between Wave 1 and Wave 2. Thus, the number of Demonstration cases followed at Wave 2 decreased by 1 and the number followed at the Comparison site increased by 1.

differences among study participants, and the overall sample was fairly representative of other children in treatment.

One of the major challenges to longitudinal research is the retention of participants throughout the course of the study. Loss of cases can limit the ability or "power" to detect results. Moreover, differential attrition (or site differences in the types of cases lost over time) can bias the analysis and interpretation of outcomes. Various strategies were utilized to retain participants in the Evaluation. Site Coordinators phoned families after the first interview to assess satisfaction and address any problems. Respondents were paid for their time, and transportation and child care were provided at no cost. Two follow-up letters were sent after each wave of data collection. The first was sent within 3 months of the last interview and the second just prior to the next interview. The 3-month letter capitalized on the United States Postal Service's free service of reporting a change of address within 3 months of a move. The 6-month letter reminded the family that the Site Coordinator would be contacting them soon to schedule the next series of interviews. Both letters provided an opportunity to thank the participants, remind them of the importance of their continued participation, and determine whether they had changed their address or phone number.

Site staff were instructed to persist in efforts to contact families. If a family moved from one Project catchment area to another, the case was transferred to the receiving site office. If a family moved out of all Project catchment areas, efforts were made to conduct interviews over the telephone. Military families who moved were tracked via the World-Wide Locator Service and other available databases. With information and consent obtained at recruitment, friends and relatives were contacted when participants could not be found. Families who could not be located or who refused to provide any information at Wave 2 were considered "circumstantial" refusals (Navratil, Green, Loeber, & Lahey, 1994) and pursued at Wave 3, 1 year after entry into the study. Only families that specifically requested never to be contacted again were dropped permanently from follow-up efforts.

The bottom of Table 2.1 shows the success of the retention efforts. Attrition from the Project was minimal and at the same rate statistically at both sites. Of the 984 families who completed Wave 1, 92% participated at Wave 2, and 83% at Wave 3. These figures include families who provided minimal data on service utilization as well as those who provided additional diagnostic information. Completion rates are still favorable when the more stringent criterion is used, that is, when diagnostic data necessary for assessing mental health outcomes were also obtained; overall, 84% of families completed Wave 2 and 73% completed Wave 3 by this criterion.

These findings compare very favorably to retention rates reported by others (Capaldi & Patterson, 1987).

Data Collection

Logistics

Each research participant was asked to participate in three data collection waves over a 1-year period. Wave 1 was conducted within 30 days of entry into mental health services and the Project. Wave 2 and Wave 3 followed at 6-month intervals. Each wave included a brief telephone interview, face-to-face diagnostic interviews, and self-report questionnaires, for which families were paid $40 per wave. Logistics associated with the face-to-face interviews were the most complex.

Project staff recruited interviewers from the sites' surrounding communities. While interviewers were laypersons, most had prior experience in working either with children or in the field of mental health. Project staff developed extensive protocols to train and monitor interviewers' performance. For example, after six training sessions, interviewers scored 10 mock interviews specially videotaped for training. Interviewers' scores were compared to those of the instrument's developer, Dr. Kay Hodges. Kappa coefficients greater than or equal to .75 indicated an acceptable level of agreement between the two sets of ratings. Only interviewers who met this criterion on at least 80% of their scored interviews advanced to the next level of training. There, successful interviewers actually conducted five videotaped pilot interviews. The Project retained only those who again met the reliability criterion—kappa GE .75 on at least 80% of the interviews. Project staff continued to monitor interviewers' performance throughout the Project by reviewing 10% of all interviews conducted. Moreover, staff provided extensive feedback to interviewers and site coordinators, and required remedial training of interviewers who fell below the established criterion.

Sources of Outcome Data

The Project developed comprehensive instrumentation to generate a multidimensional profile of children's mental health. A comprehensive profile includes measures of children's psychopathology and competence, as well as factors that can affect children's treatment success, such as satisfaction with services (Furey & Basili, 1988; Kalman, 1983; Kazdin, 1980; Lebow, 1987; Pascoe & Attkisson, 1983) and family functioning (McCubbin, 1987). Many standardized instruments used by other researchers were used or adapted for the Project. Additional instruments were developed when needed to provide more complete information. Each wave of data collection included independent, semistructured diagnostic interviews of the parent and child, behavioral checklists, family well-being scales, and demographic and background information. At follow-up, data on client satisfaction with services were also obtained.

Semistructured Diagnostic Interview. Most diagnostic interviews for children were originally designed for use with adults. The Child Assessment Schedule (CAS) (Hodges, Kline, Stern, Cytryn, & McKnew, 1982) and its version for parents, the P-CAS, were developed to fill the growing need for standardized clinical diagnostic tools appropriate for children. While the interview was originally designed for children 7–12 years old, its most recent versions have been successfully used for adolescents (Kashani, Orvaschel, Rosenberg, & Reid, 1989; Runyan, Everson, Edelsohn, Hunter, & Coulter, 1988).

The interview generates two types of clinical information—problems related to specific "content areas" and diagnoses. Content areas are: school, friends, activities and hobbies, family, fears, worries and anxieties, self-image, mood (particularly sadness), somatic complaints, expression of anger, and thought disorder. Items in each area are scored, after which respondents are asked about onset and duration for items positively endorsed. These inquiries are made after item endorsement to enhance the reliability of responses (Hodges & Cools, 1990). The arrangement of items emulates a traditional clinical interview organized around topics of natural conversation.

Items related to diagnoses are interspersed within content areas and generate diagnoses corresponding to the *Diagnostic and Statistical Manual of Mental Disorders*, 3rd edition—revised (DSM-III-R) (American Psychiatric Association, 1987). Diagnoses that can be made reliably are: attention-deficit disorder, conduct disorder, oppositional disorder, major depressive episode, dysthymia, obsessive–compulsive disorder, separation anxiety, overanxious disorder, and phobic disorders.

The interview generates categorical data (e.g., type of diagnosis) as well as several quantitative measures of total psychopathology, content area problems, and diagnostic symptom complexes. The total pathology score is the sum of the total number of items endorsed by the child and indicates the child's overall level of symptoms. Content area scores are the sums of the endorsed items within each area. (Content scores are not generated for activities or thought disorder [see Hodges & Saunders, 1989].) Diagnostic symptom scales are the sums of endorsed items associated with the various diagnostic categories.

In order to extend the interview to a slightly older population and capture a wider range of diagnostic information, items were added to the interview to indicate when eating disorder, substance abuse, psychosis, hypomania, or posttraumatic stress disorder (PTSD) might be a problem. Modules from the Diagnostic Interview Schedule for Children (Shaffer, Garland, Gould, & Fisher, 1988; Shaffer et al., 1989) were used to diagnose eating disorders, substance abuse disorders, psychosis, and hypomania. A module from the Diagnostic Interview for Children and Adolescents— Revised (Reich & Welner, 1990) was used to diagnose PTSD.

Symptoms alone cannot fully describe mental health status or explain service need. Thus, two Level of Functioning (LOF) scales were completed by Project interviewers on the basis of information from the face-to-face interviews with children and parents: the Child and Adolescent Functional Assessment Scale (CAFAS) (Hodges, 1990; Hodges, Bickman, Ring-Kurtz, & Reiter, 1992) and the Global Level of Functioning (GLOF) (Hodges, 1990).

The CAFAS (Hodges, 1990) was adapted for the Project from the North Carolina Functional Assessment Scale (NCFAS) (Langmeyer, as cited by Hodges et al., 1992). It is a rating instrument used to measure functioning in five psychosocial areas: role performance, thinking, behavior toward self and others, moods and emotions, and substance use. Two scales that seek to characterize caretaker support are also rated. Each psychosocial area receives an impairment rating of average, mild, moderate, or severe. The CAFAS yields a score for each of these subscales. It also generates an age-appropriate total score that reflects the child's lowest level of functioning in the last 30 days across all five psychosocial areas.

The GLOF is an adaptation of the Children's Global Assessment Scale (CGAS) (Shaffer et al., 1983), the most widely recognized LOF instrument for children. The LOF rating scale used in Axis V of the DSM-III-R was based on the CGAS and the adult scale (GAS) (Endicott, Spitzer, Fleiss, & Cohen, 1976), from which the CGAS was developed. The GLOF was developed because the CGAS is intended for use by highly trained clinicians. The GLOF allowed our trained interviewers to make global assessments of LOF on the basis of information they elicited from the interviews.

Behavioral Checklists. The Project also used behavior rating scales to supplement the diagnostic data. These scales have many advantages. They generate age- and gender-specific profiles that can be normed to the general population of youth. They include measures of psychopathology as well as competence, identify behaviors that occur infrequently and thus are likely to be missed by in vivo measures, have forms available for multiple respondents familiar with the child's behavior in various settings, and are inexpensive to administer and easy to complete (Achenbach & Edelbrock, 1983).

Several forms of the Child Behavior Checklist (CBCL) (Achenbach, 1991) were used in the Project: the CBCL, completed by all parents; the Youth Self-Report (YSR) (Achenbach & Edelbrock, 1987), completed by children 12 and older; and the Teacher Report Form (TRF) (Edelbrock & Achenbach, 1984). In the CBCL, 20 items generate three subscale scores that indicate the child's level of competence in activities, social relations, and school. These scores are plotted on one of six profiles, depending on the child's age (4–5 years, 6–11 years, or 12–16 years) and sex. The remaining 118 items comprise the behavior problem scales.

The YSR was designed to obtain a self-report from 11- to 18-year-olds on their personal problems and competencies. In addition, items that tap social desirability are included. The format parallels that of the CBCL. For children of ages 11–16, norms are available to compare YSR and CBCL responses and individual and sample scores with those derived from normative samples of nonreferred youth. The Project used the YSR for youth of ages 12–17 years.

The TRF is quite similar in format and item content to the CBCL. In place of the social competence profile on the parent form, the TRF uses an adaptive functioning profile that reflects the child's work habits and level of academic performance, the degree of the teacher's familiarity with the child, and the child's general happiness. Information on grade point average, achievement test scores, and special class placement is requested. The behavior problem checklist, like that for the parent form, generates a number of factorially developed scales spanning a broad range of child psychopathologies. These profiles also differ according to the age and sex of the child, respecting the changing nature of psychopathology across the developmental span of childhood and adolescence.

The Teacher-Child Rating Scale (T-CRS) (Hightower et al., 1986) is a brief instrument designed to measure problem behaviors and competencies at school. It was developed from two questionnaires used in the Primary Mental Health Project (Cowen, 1980): the Classroom Adjustment Rating Scale (Lorion, Cowen, & Caldwell, 1975) and the Health Resources Inventory (Gesten, 1976). Part II of the T-CRS, which assesses competencies, was used by the Project and includes the following subscales: Frustration Tolerance, Assertive Social Skills, Task Orientation, and Peer Social Skills.

Finally, the Self-Perception Profile (SPP) (Harter, 1985) was selected to measure self-evaluative processes related to social competence. The SPP, a revision of the Perceived Competence Scale (Harter, 1982), was developed to address conceptual and psychometric concerns with other self-evaluative measures. Completed by children of ages 8–17, the SPP generates five subscales: Scholastic Competence, Athletic Competence, Social Acceptance, Physical Appearance, and Behavioral Conduct. The Adolescent (A-SPP) version administered to youth of ages 12–17 generates three additional subscales: Close Friendship, Romantic Appeal, and Job Competence.

Family Well-Being Measures. Family assessment measures take a variety of forms that include observational coding schemes, global rating scales, structured interviews, experimental tasks, and self-report measures. Given the Project's limitation in interview time, five self-report questionnaires were used to measure two types of family variables—global family functioning and family stressors and resources.

Global family functioning measures served two purposes. First, such measures provided a context of general family environment that may affect child functioning and participation in treatment. Second, family functioning itself was considered an outcome because it may change as a result of participation in treatment. Two instruments were used to assess global family functioning: the Family Assessment Device (FAD) (Epstein, Baldwin, & Bishop, 1983; Miller, Epstein, Bishop, & Keitner, 1985) and the Family Index of Regenerativity and Adaptation (FIRA) (McCubbin, 1987).

The FAD is based on the McMaster Model of Family Functioning that views families as interactional systems (Epstein et al., 1983). The 60-item instrument is designed to be completed by all family members of ages 12 and older. The FAD generates six subscales that measure aspects of family life considered crucial for healthy family functioning—Problem Solving, Communication, Roles, Affective Responsiveness, Affective Involvement, and Behavior Control—and a General Functioning Scale.

The FIRA was designed to operationalize part of the resources component of the Double ABCX model of family adjustment (McCubbin & Patterson, 1983), portions of which were adapted for military families (McCubbin, Patterson, & Lavee, 1983). FIRA subscales used for the Project included social support, friend and relative support, and a family index of coherence.

Family stressors and sources of support were measured by three instruments: the Family Inventory of Life Events (FILE) (McCubbin, Hamilton, & Patterson, 1981), the Family Resource Scale (FRS) (Dunst & Leet, 1987), and the Burden of Care Questionnaire (BCQ) (Brannan, Heflinger, & Bickman, 1994). Each was completed by the primary caretaker. An adolescent version of the FILE was also completed by youth of ages 12–17. Additional items that measure stressors were also included in the background and demographic information form developed by Project staff.

The FILE is designed to record the normative and nonnormative life events and changes in a family. Of the 71 items, 34 refer to events that are chronic and that generate a prolonged amount of stress (e.g., spouse/parent separation or divorce, child becoming seriously ill or injured, family member losing a job). The others refer to events within the preceding year. Each item is worded to reflect a change of sufficient magnitude to require some adjustment in the regular pattern of interaction among family members. Thus, the FILE assesses the "pile-up" of life events as conceptualized by the Double ABCX model (McCubbin & Patterson, 1983).

The FRS is a 31-item questionnaire that measures parental perceptions of the adequacy of resources (e.g., time, energy, money) available in their household. Availability of resources has been correlated with personal well-being (Dunst, 1986a) and parents' commitment to follow through with treatment recommended for their child (Dunst, 1986b).

The BCQ is a 42-item questionnaire based on the work of previous researchers (Grad & Sainsbury, 1968; Hoenig & Hamilton, 1967; Montgomery, Stull, & Bagatta, 1985; Thompson & Doll, 1982). Seven areas of burden are assessed: disruption of family life and relationships, demands on time, negative mental and physical health effects, financial strain, disruption of social life, worry and emotional strain, and embarrassment. Moreover, objective and subjective dimensions of burden are measured. Respondents are asked to indicate how much of a problem burdensome occurrences or feelings were in the prior 6 months. The respondent is also instructed to indicate whether the burden is more or less of a problem since the child entered treatment.

Satisfaction Scales. The continuum-of-care model was expected to enhance client satisfaction (see Figure 1.1). The continuum of care established by the Demonstration involved a variety of programs with numerous components. This multiplicity made the assessment of consumer (parent and child) satisfaction a more complicated procedure. An overall, posttest evaluation of client satisfaction could not adequately address each of these experiences. On the basis of the "component theory of evaluation" described by Bickman (1985) and Banspach (1986), separate instruments were developed to assess client satisfaction with each component of care.

Demographic and Background Information. Primary caretakers provided additional information such as family members' economic and educational status, the child's school status and involvement with the juvenile justice system, service costs, service utilization, military background, parental absence, and family mobility.

Provider Surveys. The Project developed a survey to be completed by the children's service providers at follow-ups. At Wave 2 and Wave 3, providers described their contacts with the child and family and recorded their diagnosis of the child's mental health. Surveys were mailed to up to two providers for each child. (These data are not presented in this book.)

List of Outcome Measures. The following instruments were used to measure mental health outcomes:

- Child Assessment Schedule (CAS)
- Child and Adolescent Functional Assessment Scale (CAFAS)
- Global Level of Functioning (GLOF)
- Child Behavior Checklist (CBCL)
- Youth Self-Report (YSR)
- Teacher Report Form (TRF)
- Teacher–Child Rating Scale (T-CRS)
- Self-Perception Profile (SPP)
- Family Assessment Device (FAD)
- Family Index of Regenerativity and Adaptation (FIRA)
- Family Inventory of Life Events (FILE)
- Family Resource Scale (FRS)
- Burden of Care Questionnaire (BCQ)
- Satisfaction scales
- Demographic and background information
- Provider surveys

Data Management

Producing and managing a complex and large database was one of the challenges of the Outcome Study. Data Management staff held two broad objectives: to monitor adherence to the evaluation design of the Project and to ensure the quality of the data for reporting and analysis. While a variety of means were developed to accomplish each of these goals, two are discussed in detail—a specialized tracking system and comprehensive protocols for data cleaning.

Tracking System

The tracking system contained a variety of information about the families and children in treatment, including the status of cases and the instruments that participants completed. This specialized database enabled staff to make early identification of problems, such as unacceptably high levels of attrition, and solve them. Another function of the tracking system was to protect the identity of respondents. This protection was achieved, in part, through a two-number identification system. Field site staff assigned each family a unique "contact number" for use at the site.

Upon receipt of case materials, however, Data Management staff replaced the site-assigned number with its own unique identifier. Thus, information could not be linked with personal records maintained at the site, except through Data Management.

Data Cleaning Protocols

At the outset, it was known that the Project would generate a comprehensive database on children's mental health services. Three waves of data collection generated 107 data files containing over 17,000 variables for 984 clients. Recognizing the need for accurate as well as comprehensive information, staff developed strategies for reviewing cases before and after data entry.

Before data entry, a two-layer review process was implemented. Site Coordinators checked case materials before shipment to Data Management staff, who then checked the information and provided written feedback to sites. Additionally, special data entry programs were designed to define the acceptable codes that could be entered for each question. Data were entered twice, with verification, ensuring that the two sets of data for a given case corresponded before another case was entered. After data entry, cleaning programs were applied to check for a predefined range of problems, including appropriate branching across items. These checks were primarily within-instrument and within-wave. Across-instrument comparisons (e.g., whether male respondents of the YSR responded to items about menstruation in the CAS) and across-wave checks (e.g., whether age increased by more than 1 year between consecutive waves) were not conducted. Because data cleaning is an ongoing process, analysts were given special forms with which they could report problems that extended beyond the scope of the general cleaning plan. Measures such as these have helped ensure the integrity of the database and the contribution it can make to the field of children's mental health services research.

THE COST/UTILIZATION STUDY

Unlike data on mental health outcomes, data on service utilization and costs[2] were compiled from a variety of secondary sources. Thus, some issues relevant for the Outcome Study, such as participant recruitment, were irrelevant for the C/U Study. Moreover, the C/U Study was based on

---

[2]We acknowledge the distinction between "costs" and "charges." Chapter 7 explains the implications of this distinction.

the Evaluation Sample as well as all children treated and all children eligible for treatment within the catchment areas. This section describes the sources of data for the C/U Study and the modifications made to generate a database appropriate for cost and utilization analyses.

Data from the Demonstration Site

The Rumbaugh Clinic's Management Information System (MIS) described services provided during the Demonstration period. It included three data files: the service transaction file, the diagnostic transaction file, and the demographic file. The *service transaction file* contained over a half million transactions, with each transaction containing over 50 variables. This transactional data file recorded utilization information for every treatment encounter facilitated by the Rumbaugh Clinic. This information included the specific service and the number of service units received, the date of service, and the date the transaction was recorded in the MIS. The *diagnostic transaction file* contained almost 100,000 transactions with over 30 variables. It included the date of diagnosis and diagnostic summaries for all axes of the DMS-III-R for principal, primary, and secondary diagnoses. Unlike the other MIS data files, the *demographic file* was not transactional; it contained one record of 60 variables for each of the over 8000 clients. This file contained age, race, and gender of the children, their caretakers, and their CHAMPUS sponsors.

The MIS, however, lacked information on the costs of services provided. Deriving these costs required additional calculations based on the Unit Cost Findings Report of Cardinal Mental Health Group, Inc. (see Chapter 1 for more detail on Cardinal). This report describes total expenditures on services in 20 categories. The first step in producing per-unit costs, therefore, was to group transactions into service categories. This grouping was done using two variables: the service delivery program (e.g., in-home services, contracted services, case management) and the specific service (e.g., psychotherapy, hospitalization, intake and assessment) received. From these data, 20 service types could be matched to those used in Cardinal's report. Once transactions were grouped, the per-unit cost for services in each category was determined by dividing total expenditures in that category by the total number of services received. It is important to note that some services (e.g., inpatient rounds) were included in descriptions of costs but not of utilization. Other services not considered direct (e.g., outpatient care coordination) were excluded from descriptions of utilization and costs.

Per-unit costs as reported in Cardinal's Unit Cost Findings Report for fiscal year 1992 were used to calculate the costs of services delivered. To assure that the unit costs used were as accurate as possible, Project staff worked closely with Cardinal's Unit Cost Finding subcommittee by attending committee meetings and continually consulting with committee members. Fiscal-year unit costs for 1992 were applied to fiscal years 1991 and 1993 because 1992 was the year for which complete data were available. Because of the lack of data, valuing services in 1991 and 1993 using the 1992 per-unit costs produced estimates of total expenditures that were lower than actual expenditures. This discrepancy required that per-unit costs for these other years be inflated by roughly 24% in each year.

Data from the Comparison Site

The primary source of utilization data for the Comparison site was the records of the CHAMPUS system. CHAMPUS data are maintained at Brooks Air Force Base and were accessed via the Medical Analysis Support System. Over 60,000 records were downloaded to the Project's computers. These data describe the mental health services financed by CHAMPUS for all individuals living in the three catchment areas for fiscal years 1988–1993.

The CHAMPUS database provides information on all claims filed with CHAMPUS. For families with other insurance, CHAMPUS requires that all other insurance be used prior to filing CHAMPUS claims. While services paid for out of pocket by beneficiaries or by other insurers may not appear in the files, there is financial incentive for individuals to file claims on services paid for by other insurers prior to accessing CHAMPUS benefits.[3] Payments made to other insurers (by beneficiaries for their cost-sharing requirements) and payments made by other insurers count toward the individual child's or the family's CHAMPUS cost-sharing requirements and the "catastrophic cap" on personal expenditures.[4]

Services in the CHAMPUS database are grouped into two categories: professional and institutional. Separate databases are maintained for each.

---

[3]Project staff acknowledge that, especially in the military environment, there may be disincentives to file mental health claims. These disincentives may include stigmatization of the family, fear of consequences for the sponsor, and concern for the confidentiality of the child's records.

[4]However, there are no records in the CHAMPUS database of services provided or payments made after CHAMPUS benefits were used/exhausted. For example, if at some point further inpatient services were denied by the reviewing organization, in many states Medicaid could be accessed through the Ribicoff Amendment, which allows children in out-of-home treatment to be considered a family of one for purposes of determining financial assets. A second similar example is the transfer to a state-funded hospital bed after CHAMPUS benefits have been exhausted. The Demonstration collected payments from other insurers prior to the use of Demonstration funds and the Demonstration paid for all services once the CHAMPUS benefit began; no services were covered by Medicaid or by state funds.

The Composite Professional Services Record (CPR) contains transactions for professional services; the Composite Institutional Record (CIR) contains transactions for institutional services. Transactions in the CPR and the CIR contain extensive information on clients and the care they have received. Each record is identified by a patient identification code—a combination of the military sponsor's Social Security number and the child's year of birth. The code also includes information on the client's relationship to the sponsor. A "client-level" database for the CPR and the CIR was developed by grouping transactions that pertained to the same individual.

Each transaction in the CIR and CPR notes the amount billed for each service and the source of payments (government, individual, or third-party payer). There is some redundancy in the CIR and CPR. The CIR includes records of payment for institutional and professional services rendered to children in inpatient facilities. The professional services are also recorded in the CPR. To avoid double-counting professional services, redundant records were removed from the CIR and coded in the CPR as outpatient visits.

Each record in the CPR and CIR contains providers' diagnostic codes based on the *International Classification of Diseases*, 9th edition (World Health Organization, 1978). All records in the files attached to a psychiatric diagnosis were selected. The CIR contained as many as five diagnoses[5] per transaction, and a record was selected from it when any of the diagnoses were psychiatric in nature.[6]

Each record in the CPR also contained the Physician's Current Procedural Terminology (CPT) code describing the services provided. Each service was assigned a service category. Unless a CPT code was provided, records in the CIR described care provided in either a psychiatric hospital or an RTC.[7] A small minority of CIR records contained CPT codes, which were assigned using the same scheme as was used for the CPR.

A single transaction in the CIR could have referred to multiple days of hospitalization (or care in an RTC). The beginning and ending day of the hospital stay was recorded in the file, creating a record for each day of hospitalization or RTC care.[8] Records were also "bundled" in the CPR. In particular, outpatient services received on different days were sometimes combined into a single transaction. The record in the CHAMPUS file for

[5]The additional diagnoses were provided when the bill represented care from more than one provider during a stay in a hospital or RTC.
[6]V-codes were not classified as diagnoses.
[7]Hospitalization can be distinguished from the RTC using an additional variable, "basis for care," provided in the CIR file.
[8]The day of admission and the day of discharge were counted as hospital days.

such a transaction did not record the day on which each service was received. Rather, it recorded the date services began and ended. This characteristic of data recording involved only a minority of transactions (16%), but for those cases it was impossible to determine the exact dates on which services were received. When a transaction recorded services received on multiple days, Project staff counted half as occurring on the beginning date and half on the ending date.

Similarly, it was impossible to determine the number of services received on a given day (e.g., to determine whether an individual had two outpatient visits on a single day). This inability arose because different providers might bill in different units. For an hour of outpatient therapy, one provider might bill for a single 1-hour unit, while another might bill for four 15-minute intervals. Because of these differences, all services of a given type on a given day were collapsed into a single unit. Where days were the natural unit for calculating length of service (e.g., hospitalization), grouping services received on the same day was inconsequential. For services like outpatient therapy, however, grouping services of the same type that occurred on the same day affected analyses and discussion about service use and cost. The unit of these services was no longer visits but service encounters—days on which these services were received.

Other Sources of Data

CHAMPUS System for the Fort Bragg Catchment Area

While CHAMPUS files were the main source of data for the Comparison site, they also provided supplemental information for the Demonstration site. The CHAMPUS contract with the fiscal intermediary for the Fort Bragg catchment area, Blue Cross/Blue Shield of South Carolina, did not require CHAMPUS to remove claims for services rendered during the Demonstration period; thus, it was possible for claims submitted by local providers to be paid through CHAMPUS contrary to the design of the Demonstration. Analyses of these data revealed that during the Demonstration period, 1165 children received services that were paid by CHAMPUS.

Fort Campbell Management Information System

Fort Campbell was an early implementer of the Gateway to Care system. As part of Gateway, services were provided within the military treatment facility (post hospital) and thus outside the CHAMPUS system. Consequently, CHAMPUS data understated the volume of services Comparison site children received. However, service utilization records were maintained in an MIS, and this information was included in some of the analyses discussed below.[9]

Evaluation Sample

Our subcontract did not allow for a concentrated effort to collect data on care received outside the mental health system. However, the Evaluation Sample provided information on services received from alternative care and support systems such as the child's school, the general medical community, religious professionals, and juvenile justice authorities, as well as self-help efforts and support provided by family and friends. Parents also reported information about their own employment problems, work hours and wages lost, and the monetary value of damage inflicted on persons and property by their child because of emotional problems. This information shed light on costs incurred outside the direct mental health service system.

Records Review

Reviews of medical records also were conducted at the Demonstration and Comparison sites to augment primary data sources. At the Demonstration site, nearly 300 records were reviewed to assess the reliability of the Rumbaugh Clinic's MIS. Cases from the early part of the Demonstration period were emphasized because of Rumbaugh Clinic staff reports that the MIS was not functioning properly then. Nonetheless, comparisons of the record review data and the MIS found that the MIS was not missing significant data. At the Comparison site, Gateway redirected children to services on post rather than in the community. These services and costs were not part of CHAMPUS data files. The records review generated utilization data for those children not already in the CHAMPUS database who entered the Project during the period July 1990 to June 1993. Data for 195 Fort Stewart participants and 213 Fort Campbell cases who had completed at least one follow-up wave of data collection were added to the Project's C/U database.

State Records on CHAMPUS-Eligible Children Hospitalized in Tennessee

Because of Fort Campbell's location along the Kentucky–Tennessee border, some families in its catchment area were eligible for services that were unavailable to families at Fort Bragg and Fort Stewart. The State of

[9]Fort Stewart did not maintain an MIS.

Table 2.2. Percentage of Transactions
Posted by Quarter for the CHAMPUS
System and the Rumbaugh Clinic
Management Information System

Time lag	Demonstration MIS	CHAMPUS
3 Months	94%	58%
6 Months	97%	83%
9 Months	99%	87%
12 Months	100%	93%

Tennessee incurs the costs of inpatient treatment in public and private hospitals for children in custody. Anecdotal information suggested that some families chose to reside in Tennessee and avail themselves of State-funded care. For a time, the military treatment facility commander at Fort Campbell encouraged families to use this feature of Tennessee's treatment system rather than use their CHAMPUS benefits. Records for these children would not appear in the CHAMPUS and MIS databases. State officials provided information on the number of CHAMPUS-eligible children they served in fiscal year 1991 and the duration of services.[10] Given the lack of information for other years, the fiscal year 1991 data were assumed to be the same for succeeding years in the Demonstration period.

Comparability of Data between Sites

To ensure complete and comparable data sets, only services provided between October 1, 1990, and September 30, 1993, are described in this book. However, because of the time lag in posting claims, MIS and CHAMPUS records were downloaded through May 1994. Table 2.2 presents the proportion of claims that appeared within various time periods for the Demonstration and Comparison sites. Note, for example, that 83% of CHAMPUS claims appeared in the CHAMPUS database within 6 months[11] of the delivery of the corresponding service. This partial entry does not mean that the CHAMPUS database was only 83% complete. Since virtually all services were received more than a year prior to the last download, the database used by the Project contained nearly 100% of services received. Most services appeared almost immediately in the MIS;

[10]This information comes from reports accessed by personnel at the Mid Cumberland Community Health Agency in Clarksville, Tennessee. Additional years were requested, but they could not be provided by the State.
[11]Of those services that are not posted within 6 months, 85% are outpatient therapy.

Table 2.3. Combined Service Categories for CHAMPUS and MIS Data
Used in Utilization and Cost Determination, Ranked by Restrictiveness

Service category	Description
Acute inpatient care	Psychiatric hospitalization
Residential treatment center	See footnote a
Periodic inpatient care[b]	Emergency room or hospital visit without admission due to psychiatric-related problem
Intermediate residential[c]	Therapeutic home, therapeutic group home
Intermediate nonresidential[c]	In-home services, after school program, latency partial hospitalization, day treatment
Clinical case management[c]	See footnote a
Outpatient treatment	See footnote a
Psychiatric/psychological assessment and evaluation	Intake/assessment, neuropsychological evaluation, and intelligence testing, etc.
Medical evaluation	Pharmacology management, EKG, urinalysis

[a]The description is redundant with the service category.
[b]This category does not include hospital rounds, admission, or discharge.
[c]Service available only at the Demonstration site.

virtually all services (94%) had been entered within 3 months of their delivery. Data collection continued for 7 months following the end of the Demonstration period. Thus, the database on services received during that period should be complete for both sites.

The primary sources of utilization data were different for the two sites; therefore, special efforts were undertaken to create comparability of data. Services of the same type that occurred on the same day were collapsed into one unit for both sites.[12] Thus, the unit of observation was no longer a visit, but a service encounter. It was also crucial that services be aggregated the same way for the two data systems. CHAMPUS used the standardized CPT codes, while the developers of the Demonstration's MIS constructed their own system. The MIS contained over 300 service codes, with an additional code that placed services into different program groups. Equating the two coding schemes was done by grouping all services in each system into nine service categories. These categories are listed in Table 2.3 and ranked in order from the most to the least restrictive service.

[12]As noted above, it was necessary to do so for the Comparison data and was done for the Demonstration data as well.

SUMMARY AND CONCLUSIONS

This chapter described the methods used to collect and manage the data associated with the Outcome and Cost/Utilization studies. A comprehensive database was required for each study to address adequately its specific research questions. The material presented here highlights the volumes of data the Project made available and the special efforts that were taken to ensure that the information on which the studies' results were based was reliable and valid.

3

Description of
the Evaluation Sample

This chapter describes the 984 children and families who comprised the Evaluation Sample of the Mental Health Outcome Study. Data are presented to show the comparability of children and families at the Demonstration and Comparison sites at the time the Evaluation began. Site differences with regard to differential attrition during the course of the Evaluation are also addressed. Finally, information on the overall sample's representativeness of other families and children who have mental or emotional disorders is also provided.

SAMPLE CHARACTERISTICS AND SITE
COMPARISONS AT INTAKE

The Outcome Study was quasi-experimental; participants were not randomly assigned to the Demonstration or Comparison site. Thus, the evaluation of the effectiveness of treatment required the assessment of site differences prior to the onset of treatment. Otherwise, apparent treatment effects might actually be the result of initial group differences. This section reports the extent to which the Demonstration and Comparison sites recruited equivalent samples in three areas: child and family background, the child's mental health status, and family well-being.

Child and Family Background

Demographics

Demographic profiles of children in treatment may relate directly or indirectly to treatment effectiveness. Thus, initial demographic differences between sites could bias the analysis of mental health outcomes. For example, gender differences in the types of problems children experience have been observed. Females have higher prevalence rates of depression and report a greater number of depressive symptoms than males (Elliott, Huizinga, & Menard, 1989). Smaller treatment effects have been found in samples that include greater proportions of males (Casey & Berman, 1985). Younger clients seem to benefit more from treatment than do adolescents (Weisz & Weiss, 1987). Family background may also influence mental health outcomes. Disadvantaged families, for example, may lack the knowledge, motivation, financial resources, or trust in the medical community (Dryfoos, 1990) to derive full benefit from formal services.

Table 3.1 summarizes demographic profiles of children and families at the Demonstration and Comparison sites. There were no significant site differences in children's gender, age, race, or family structure. Families at the Demonstration site, however, had significantly higher levels of education and, relatedly, income.

Military Background

The military status of the families at the two sites is shown in Table 3.2. The Demonstration site was similar to the Comparison site on most variables. The majority of families (about 70%) had a primary caretaker who was currently active in the military. Nearly 20% of families had a primary caretaker who had served actively but was retired or otherwise discharged from service when entering the Evaluation. Only about 10% of households did not have a primary caretaker with military experience.[1]

Sites differed significantly as to the branch of the military in which participants were currently serving or had previously served. The Demonstration sample included a greater proportion of Air Force personnel; the Comparison site, a greater proportion of Army personnel. This difference was expected, since the catchment area for Fort Bragg also included Pope Air Force Base and more Air Force families were therefore available to be recruited there than at the Comparison site.

Family disruption was also examined with regard to whether a pri-

[1]The eligibility for CHAMPUS for this group of children depended on an absent military sponsor (e.g., a divorced father who no longer lived at home).

Table 3.1. Demographic Profiles at Intake
for 984 Families in the Evaluation Sample

Characteristic	Demonstration (N = 574)	Comparison (N = 410)	p(α)[a]
Gender			
Male	62%	64%	.53
Female	38%	36%	
Mean age	11.0 years	11.4 years	.07
Race			
White	72%	70%	.18
African-American	18%	16%	
Other	10%	14%	
Family structure			
Two biological parents	48%	44%	.07
Blended[b]	30%	37%	
Single head of household	12%	11%	
Other	10%	8%	
Education			
High school or less	13%	23%	.00
Some college	58%	54%	
BA/BS	15%	15%	
Postgraduate	14%	8%	
Income			
< $20,000	28%	36%	.02
$20,000–$40,000	57%	52%	
> $40,000	15%	12%	

[a]Based on χ^2 for nominal (categorical) variables or one-way ANOVA for continuous variables.
[b]"Blended" is defined as a family with one biological parent and one step, adoptive, or foster parent.

mary caretaker had been deployed in the 6 months before intake to the study, the amount of time the caretaker was away from home because of military duties, and the number of times the caretaker had ever been reassigned while living with the child participant. A significantly greater proportion of caretakers at the Demonstration site (33%) had been deployed than at the Comparison site (27%). The duration of separation associated with any military duty, however, was statistically the same at both sites. Moreover, the number of reassignments families experienced was also comparable at both sites.

Involvement in Child-Serving Systems

Previous involvement in the mental health system might condition treatment effectiveness. Limited data were available that indicated the

Table 3.2. Military Profiles of Families

Characteristic	N	Demonstration	N	Comparison	$p(\alpha)^a$
Duty status					
Active	401	70.8%	291	72.0%	0.97
Nonactive	108	19.1%	74	18.3%	
Never in military	57	10.1%	39	9.7%	
TOTALS	566	100%	404	100%	
Rank					
Enlisted	423	85.1%	323	90.0%	0.07
Warrant officer	42	8.5%	19	5.3%	
Officer	32	6.4%	17	4.7%	
TOTALS	497	100%	359	100%	
Branch					
Army	428	84.7%	343	94.5%	<0.01
Air Force	68	13.5%	12	3.3%	
Navy	4	0.8%	6	1.7%	
Marines	3	0.6%	2	0.5%	
Other	2	0.4%	0	—	
TOTALS	505	100%	363	100%	
Deployed	163	33.4%	91	26.5%	0.03
Days away from home	301	58.1 days[b]	223	61.6 days[b]	0.52
Reassignments	312	2.9[c]	223	3.0[c]	0.88

[a]Based on χ^2 for nominal (categorical) variables or one-way ANOVA for continuous variables.
[b]Mean number of days away from home.
[c]Mean number of reassignments.

number of different types of service settings (e.g., psychiatric hospitalization, residential treatment center) the child had experienced prior to entry into the Project. Table 3.3 shows that prior service use[2] at the Demonstration site was slightly higher than at the Comparison site. Children at the Demonstration site also had a higher school attendance rate and were significantly less likely to have a history of arrest than children at the Comparison site.

In summary, 16 measures of child and family background were examined for site differences; 7 met the statistical criterion of $p < 0.05$. Only

[2]The "number of services" variable is based on a count of the *types* of formal mental health services previously used. It does not reflect the number of times any service was used or the duration of treatment. Additionally, 19% of children at the Demonstration site entered the Evaluation upon transition to a different level of treatment. Some services they received prior to transition were provided through the Demonstration. Thus, the transition cases may inflate somewhat the mental health service utilization data in Table 3.3.

Table 3.3. Involvement in Child-Serving Systems

Characteristic	Demonstration	Comparison	$p(\alpha)^a$
Mental health			
Prior service	52%	53%	.75
Number of services	2.1	1.8	.01
Education			
Not attending school	7%	11%	.02
Juvenile justice			
Arrested	15%	23%	<.01

[a]Based on χ^2 for nominal (categorical) variables or one-way ANOVA for continuous variables.

2 results—branch of service and whether the children had been arrested—met the more conservative Bonferroni-adjusted alpha level of $p < 0.003$ (0.05/16).[3]

Children's Mental Health Status[4]

The following tables present baseline comparisons of the Demonstration and Comparison sites on 44 mental health measures. Because a large sample size can generate differences that are significant statistically but not meaningful, effect sizes are also reported, when calculable, to show the magnitude of the difference. The Project was designed to detect effects of 0.25 SD; smaller effects were considered too small to be interpreted as clinically meaningful.[5]

Parent Report

Global Psychopathology and Competence. Seven measures broadly assessed levels of psychopathology and competence:

[3]These site differences were not used as covariates in the outcome analysis. To do so would have further complicated an already complex analysis and also exacerbated problems with missing data. Instead, every outcome analysis tested for differences at Wave 1 on the particular outcome measure being analyzed.

[4]See Chapter 2 for a discussion of all the instruments referred to in this section.

[5]According to Lampman, Durlak, and Wells (1991), the average effect size (ES) for 61 studies of child psychopathology using normal rating scales and nonbehavioral treatment was ES = 0.24.

- The number of primary diagnoses endorsed [Child Assessment Schedule for Parents (P-CAS)][6]
- The total number of diagnoses endorsed (P-CAS)[7]
- The number of diagnostic-related problems (P-CAS)
- Total problems scale score [Child Behavior Checklist (CBCL)]
- Internalizing problems scale score (CBCL)
- Externalizing problems scale score (CBCL)
- Total competence scale score (CBCL)

Table 3.4 shows that the two groups were virtually identical at Wave 1 on all measures. The CBCL mean scores on psychopathology and competence indicate that both groups fell into the low end of the clinical range, except in internalizing problems, where they were borderline. (The P-CAS, not normed on a general population of children, does not provide clinical cutoff points for total symptom scores.)

Diagnostically Related Scale Scores. Table 3.5 presents data on seven diagnostic variables from the P-CAS and eight standardized narrow-band syndrome scores from the CBCL. Both sites' narrow-band CBCL scores fell in the nonclinical range, with means below the cutoff of 67.[6] Overall, sites were similar; they differed only with regard to two diagnostic categories— dysthymia and overanxious disorder. The effect sizes for these two measures, however, fell well below the minimum standard of 0.25 SD.

Presence of Diagnosis. The presence of a diagnosis is another way to describe the Evaluation Sample. Data were available that indicated whether the children met DSM-III-R clinical criteria in any of 26 diagnostic categories. In this sample, 6 of the diagnoses were nonexistent or rare[7] and are not presented. Additional analyses were conducted on whether the children met criteria for any primary diagnosis or any diagnosis at all. Table 3.6 shows the percentages of children at each site who met DSM-III-R criteria.

Sites differed on 3 of the 20 specific diagnostic categories: posttraumatic stress disorder (PTSD) ($p = 0.01$), school phobia ($p = 0.02$), and simple phobia ($p = 0.05$). Demonstration children were roughly twice as likely as

[6]Scores that fall below the clinical range do not mean children do not need treatment. Some children in the Evaluation Sample, for example, had near-normal Total Problem Scores (scores below 60), but had a narrow-band score as high as 74. Such children could have one problem in the clinical range and nonclinical scores on most other variables.
[7]"Rare" is defined as a diagnostic category for which fewer than 10 children (roughly 1% of the total sample) met the diagnostic criteria.

Table 3.4. Global Measures of Psychopathology and Competence of Children in the Evaluation Sample[a]

Variable	Demonstration site			Comparison site			ES[b]	p(F)[c]
	Mean	SD	N	Mean	SD	N		
Psychopathology								
P-CAS								
Primary diagnoses[d]	1.50	1.37	574	1.36	1.25	410	0.10	0.10
Total diagnoses[e]	1.75	1.15	574	1.62	1.04	410	0.11	0.07
Total diagnostic endorsements	29.20	14.00	574	30.68	13.76	410	0.11	0.10
CBCL								
Total problems	65.17	10.31	522	65.17	10.49	402	0.00	0.99
Internalizing	62.14	11.97	522	62.39	11.46	402	0.02	0.75
Externalizing	64.30	10.95	522	64.01	11.45	402	0.03	0.70
Competence								
CBCL								
Total competence	36.06	7.72	426	35.93	6.37	362	0.02	0.80

[a]Not all parents completed all instruments or all items within an instrument.
[b]Effect size is the difference between Demonstration and Comparison means expressed in SDs.
[c]Univariate probability of F.
[d]Primary diagnoses included attention-deficit disorder, conduct disorder, oppositional–defiant disorder, separation anxiety, overanxious, enuresis, encopresis, major depressive, dysthymia, obsessive–compulsive, agoraphobia, social phobia, school phobia, and simple phobia.
[e]Any diagnosis includes the primary diagnosis and adjustment disorders.

Comparison children to be diagnosed phobic; Comparison children were about twice as likely as their Demonstration counterparts to be diagnosed with PTSD. The incidence of these diagnoses, however, is infrequent relative to the other diagnostic categories. None of the differences is statistically significant at the Bonferroni-adjusted probability of $p = 0.002$.

Child Report

Psychopathology and Competence. The parent-reported information on the mental health status of children revealed close similarity between the two sites at the time the study began. Site comparability of children's reports was also examined. Table 3.7 shows the mean scores on global and diagnostic measures of child-reported psychopathology and competence, as assessed by the CAS, the Youth Self-Report (YSR), and the Self-Perception Profile (SPP) for Child (C) and Adolescent (A). Of the 25 comparisons, 5 were significant, but all with effect sizes smaller than 0.25 SD.

Table 3.5. Diagnostically Related Scale Scores of Children
in the Evaluation Sample

Variable	Demonstration site (N = 574)		Comparison site (N = 410)		ES[a]	p(F)[b]
	Mean	SD	Mean	SD		
P-CAS scale scores						
Attention-deficit	7.16	4.34	7.11	4.45	0.01	0.86
Major depression	6.52	3.88	6.99	3.88	0.12	0.06
Dysthymia	6.52	4.01	7.16	3.95	0.16	0.01
Oppositional	4.44	2.78	4.47	2.84	0.01	0.88
Overanxious	2.28	1.95	2.52	1.86	0.12	0.04
Separation anxiety	1.20	1.80	1.24	1.62	0.02	0.71
Conduct disorder	1.08	1.46	1.19	1.48	0.08	0.26
CBCL						
Aggressiveness	65.02	11.30	64.82	11.64	0.02	0.79
Attention-deficit	64.81	10.30	65.07	10.67	0.03	0.70
Delinquency	64.16	9.72	64.60	9.62	0.05	0.50
Anxious/depressed	63.08	11.03	62.96	10.07	0.01	0.86
Withdrawn	61.94	10.66	62.38	10.06	0.04	0.53
Thought problems	61.37	9.52	61.03	9.60	0.04	0.59
Social problems	60.84	9.80	61.19	9.58	0.04	0.58
Somatic complaints	59.39	10.05	59.57	9.80	0.06	0.79

[a]Effect size is the difference between Demonstration and Comparison means expressed in
SDs.
[b]Univariate probability of F.

Presence of Diagnosis. The Demonstration and Comparison sites
were also compared on 19 measures of the presence of any, primary, or
specific diagnosis at intake, as shown in Table 3.8. There was only one
significant difference: Social phobia was more common at the Demonstration site. One significant finding, however, would be expected by chance
alone.

Teacher Report

Sites were compared on the basis of teachers' perceptions of the
children. The data in Table 3.9 support the weight of the evidence thus far
shown: The mental health status of the two groups of children was nearly
identical when the Demonstration began. Neither the Teacher Report
Form (TRF) nor the Teacher–Child Rating Scale (T-CRS) shows any site
difference in the behavior or emotional well-being of the children.

Table 3.6. Presence of Parent-Reported Diagnoses
for Children in the Evaluation Sample

Diagnosis	Demonstration[a] (N = 574)	Comparison[a] (N = 410)	$p(\chi^2)$[b]
Oppositional–defiant	32.6%	32.2%	0.90
Attention-deficit	27.4%	28.5%	0.68
Dysthymia	22.0%	21.0%	0.71
Conduct disorder	11.9%	10.7%	0.59
Major depression	11.5%	11.0%	0.80
Enuresis	11.3%	9.0%	0.24
Adjustment disorder			
Mixed	10.6%	11.7%	0.60
With depressed mood	10.3%	8.3%	0.29
Phobia			
Social	7.1%	4.6%	0.11
Simple	7.1%	4.2%	0.05
Posttraumatic stress disorder	6.3%	10.7%	0.01
Overanxious	5.1%	3.2%	0.15
Phobia, school	4.5%	1.7%	0.02
Adjustment disorder with conduct and emotion disturbance	3.0%	3.7%	0.54
Encopresis	3.0%	3.7%	0.54
Drug dependence	2.1%	3.2%	0.29
Separation anxiety	2.1%	1.0%	0.17
Obsessive–compulsive	1.4%	1.7%	0.52
Mania	1.2%	1.5%	0.56
Schizophrenia	1.1%	0.5%	0.16
ANY PRIMARY DIAGNOSIS	73.3%	71.7%	0.57
ANY DIAGNOSIS	98.0%	96.3%	0.14

[a]Because a child can receive more than one diagnosis, the percentages total more than 100%.
[b]Based on χ^2 for nominal (categorical) variables.

Interviewer Report

Trained interviewers, upon completing parent and child interviews, rated the child's level of functioning on the Global Level of Functioning (GLOF) and the Child and Adolescent Functional Assessment Scale (CAFAS). Both scales provided a global measure of functioning; the latter also provides measures of functioning in specific psychosocial areas. Table 3.10 shows that at intake there were three statistically significant differences between Demonstration and Comparison groups. Two of these, both CAFAS scores, show greater impairment among the children at the Demonstration site than at the Comparison site. However, the GLOF shows less

Table 3.7. Child-Reported Psychopathology and Competence

Variable	Demonstration site			Comparison site			ES[a]	p(F)[b]
	Mean	SD	N	Mean	SD	N		
Global measures								
CAS (8–17 years)								
Primary diagnoses	0.93	1.24	384	0.96	1.20	291	0.02	0.74
Total diagnoses	1.29	1.20	384	1.37	1.13	291	0.07	0.33
Total diagnostic endorsements	21.31	13.02	384	23.39	12.78	291	0.16	0.04
YSR (12–17 years)								
Total problems	57.83	11.54	216	59.48	10.04	196	0.14	0.12
Internalizing	56.21	12.00	216	56.90	11.91	196	0.06	0.56
Externalizing	59.04	11.45	216	60.81	9.57	196	0.15	0.09
Total competence	40.43	14.65	212	39.60	11.90	196	0.06	0.53
Diagnosis/syndrome								
CAS								
Dysthymia	5.47	3.74	384	6.16	3.92	291	0.18	0.02
Major depression	4.98	3.78	384	5.68	3.79	291	0.19	0.02
Oppositional	3.48	2.44	384	3.66	2.31	291	0.07	0.32
Attention-deficit	2.93	2.46	384	3.40	2.40	291	0.19	0.01
Separation anxiety	1.74	2.01	384	1.71	1.90	291	0.01	0.87
Overanxious	1.67	1.82	384	1.79	1.77	291	0.07	0.39
Conduct disorder	1.04	1.70	384	0.99	1.56	291	0.03	0.70
YSR								
Delinquency	61.69	9.07	216	62.45	8.22	196	0.08	0.37
Indentity problems	59.96	8.81	115	59.75	9.28	114	0.02	0.86
Aggressiveness	59.32	8.76	216	60.10	8.91	196	0.09	0.37
Anxious/depressed	58.78	9.84	216	58.80	9.78	196	0.00	0.98
Attention-deficit	58.75	9.36	216	59.28	9.01	196	0.06	0.57
Somatic complaints	57.37	8.86	215	58.36	8.56	196	0.11	0.25
Withdrawn	57.27	7.99	216	57.69	8.47	196	0.05	0.60
Social problems	56.26	8.02	216	57.95	8.33	196	0.21	0.04
Thought problems	56.08	8.12	216	55.84	7.60	196	0.03	0.76
Self-perception								
C-SPP (8–11 years)	3.11	0.78	135	2.98	0.81	89	0.17	0.23
A-SPP (12–17 years)	2.88	0.80	226	2.78	0.80	194	0.13	0.21

[a]Effect size is the difference between Demonstration and Comparison means expressed in SDs.
[b]Univariate probability of F.

Table 3.8. Presence of Child-Reported Diagnoses Based on the CAS[a]

Variable	Demonstration (N = 384)	Comparison (N = 291)	$p(\chi^2)$[b]
Oppositional–defiant	25%	29%	0.26
Dysthymia	12%	14%	0.25
Attention-deficit	12%	10%	0.44
Conduct disorder	10%	6%	0.11
Drug dependence	8%	7%	0.53
Major depression	7%	9%	0.53
Phobia, simple	6%	9%	0.25
Posttraumatic stress disorder	6%	10%	0.08
Phobia, social	5%	1%	0.01
Adjustment disorder with conduct disturbance	4%	4%	0.89
Overanxious	3%	2%	0.25
Adjustment disorder with conduct and emotional disturbance	3%	2%	0.25
Phobia, school	3%	1%	0.10
Enuresis	3%	5%	0.13
Separation anxiety	2%	2%	0.57
Adjustment disorder with depressed mood	2%	1%	0.65
Drug abuse	1%	2%	0.28
ANY PRIMARY DIAGNOSIS	50%	53%	0.45
ANY DIAGNOSIS	72%	77%	0.16

[a]Diagnoses obtained for fewer than 10 cases in the total Evaluation Sample are not presented.
[b]Based on χ^2 for nominal (categorical) variables.

Table 3.9. Teacher-Reported Psychopathology and Competence

Variable	Demonstration site			Comparison site			ES[a]	$p(F)$[b]
	Mean	SD	N	Mean	SD	N		
TRF								
Total problems	59.81	10.64	324	60.35	10.82	197	0.05	0.58
Internalizing	56.88	10.23	324	57.91	10.63	197	0.10	0.27
Externalizing	58.81	11.40	324	58.62	11.53	197	0.02	0.86
Adaptive functioning	42.61	7.55	313	42.51	7.52	193	0.01	0.89
T-CRS								
Frustration tolerance	12.89	4.69	333	13.13	4.30	228	0.05	0.53
Assertive social skills	14.75	4.43	333	14.21	4.14	227	0.12	0.15
Task orientation	13.01	5.48	334	12.87	5.11	228	0.03	0.77
Peer social skills	14.80	4.99	334	14.52	4.81	228	0.06	0.52

[a]Effect size is the difference between Demonstration and Comparison means expressed in SDs.
[b]Univariate probability of F.

Table 3.10. Interviewer Ratings on the GLOF and CAFAS

Variable	Demonstration site			Comparison site			ES[a]	p(F)[b]
	Mean	SD	N	Mean	SD	N		
GLOF[c]	55.54	13.32	573	53.62	11.52	407	0.14	0.02
CAFAS[d]								
Role performance	14.18	9.56	574	12.83	9.03	410	0.14	0.03
Thinking	2.98	6.61	574	2.41	6.08	410	0.09	0.17
Behavior toward others/self	13.36	9.56	574	11.85	10.13	410	0.16	0.02
Moods/emotions	14.30	9.25	574	14.68	9.54	410	0.04	0.53
Substance use	2.01	5.82	573	2.22	6.27	410	0.04	0.58
Global functioning	46.83	27.43	574	44.00	25.00	410	0.10	0.10

[a]Effect size is the difference between Demonstration and Comparison means expressed in SDs.
[b]Univariate probability of F.
[c]Higher score indicates less impairment.
[d]Higher score indicates greater impairment.

impairment among Demonstration children. Note, though, that all effect sizes are again below 0.25 SD.

Family Well-Being

Change in mental health status is also a function of family factors. Researchers, clinicians, and family advocates have noted the important role the family plays, for instance, in identifying mental health problems and seeking treatment (Kazdin, 1989). Moreover, the family's economic and social resources, its ability to cope with stress, and the quality of the relationships among family members (e.g., McCubbin, 1987) can influence the mental health of its members and their chance for recovery.

Table 3.11 shows various measures of the emotional and physical well-being of the family. Of the ten measures considered, three indicate significant site differences. Families at the Comparison site experienced more stressful life events than those at the Demonstration site in areas such as family relations, finances, and illness. Compared to those at the Demonstration site, they also reported fewer material and emotional resources or greater problems associated with the absence of such resources as income, housing, family support, and availability of personal time. While these two differences are statistically significant, effect sizes are smaller than 0.25 SD.

The third measure, family coherence, was specifically developed for military populations (McCubbin et al., 1983). This measure estimates the control that families think they have over their future, their commitment to

Table 3.11. Family Well-Being

Variable[a]	Demonstration site			Comparison site			ES[b]	p(F)[c]
	Mean	SD	N	Mean	SD	N		
FAD								
General functioning	2.14	0.53	560	2.14	0.44	400	0.00	0.88
FILE								
Stressors	11.26	6.14	561	12.04	6.20	404	0.13	0.05
FIRA								
Coherence	54.24	9.89	403	50.80	9.51	300	0.37	<0.01
Relative and friend support	24.16	5.86	554	24.44	5.79	398	0.05	0.45
Social support index	58.82	8.55	551	58.14	7.85	398	0.08	0.22
BSI								
Symptom severity	55.54	10.97	496	56.80	10.87	361	0.11	0.10
BCQ								
Objective burden	2.01	0.93	558	2.10	0.88	397	0.10	0.12
Subjective burden								
Externalizing	2.30	0.97	543	2.28	0.89	389	0.02	0.77
Internalizing	3.36	1.04	550	3.45	1.01	395	0.09	0.18
FRS								
Resources	124.35	17.49	553	120.34	19.59	393	0.23	<0.01

[a]Instruments: (FAD) Family Assessment Device; (FILE) Family Inventory of Life Events; (FIRA) Family Index of Regenerativity and Adaptation; (BSI) Brief Symptomatology Index; (BCQ) Burden of Care Questionnaire; (FRS) Family Resource Scale.
[b]Effect size is the difference between Demonstration and Comparison means expressed in SDs.
[c]Univariate probability of F.

military life, and their belief that the military will support them in times of need. Families at the Comparison site experienced significantly greater problems in these areas than others. Both the probability value ($p \leq 0.01$) and the effect size (0.37 SD) suggest an important site difference with regard to families' beliefs about their life in the military.

Summary of Significant Site Differences at Wave 1

In this study, 129 measures of child and family background, military profile, and mental health status of the child and family at Wave 1 were examined. Of 129 comparisons, one would expect 6 to be significant by chance. A total of 23 (18%) showed statistically significant site differences, but only 3 of the 15 for which an effect size could be computed[8] also yielded an effect size greater than or equal to 0.25 SD. These variables are summarized in Table 3.12. Demonstration families had higher socio-

[8]Effect sizes can be computed for continuous variables only.

economic status, reported less stress and uncertainty, and had greater material and emotional resources available than those at the Comparison site.

Of the 129 measures referred to above, 103 were measures of the mental health status of the children at intake. Of these 103 measures, 14 (14%) suggested that the two sites differed significantly: Of the 14, 9 (64%) indicated that children at the Comparison site exhibited greater symptomatology than those at the Demonstration site; 5 (36%) suggested that the children at the Demonstration site were more severely impaired. These site differences depended on the specific diagnostic-related area considered as well as the informant who provided the information. The most consistent findings were that Comparison children tended to be more severely depressed and less phobic than those at the Demonstration site[9] None of the effect sizes associated with the mental health status of children was greater than 0.25 SD. The Evaluation Sample, particularly with regard to mental health status, was nearly identical at the two sites at the time participants entered the Project. It is therefore unlikely that any differences in outcome at later waves could be a result of initial differences between sites.

SITE COMPARABILITY OVER TIME

Bias Due to Differential Attrition[10]

Attrition does not bias outcome if relevant data are missing at random and observed at random (Rubin, 1976). Because these conditions could not be met, special efforts were taken to determine whether differential attrition affected the results of the Outcome Study. The most important outcome variables, including eight instrument totals[11] and four individualized[12] outcomes, were used in three site comparisons to assess: (1) whether

---

[9]Recall that the measures of phobia were based on the percentage of children for whom these diagnoses were rendered, not their *level* of symptomatology within these areas. Different results may have been found if mean levels of phobic symptomatology were available for comparison.

[10]See Chapter 2 for a discussion of participant recruitment and retention strategies.

[11]The eight instrument totals (numbered as in Tables 3.13–3.15) were: (1) overall outcome (1/3path. + 1/3funct. + 1/3burden); (2) CBCL pathology total; (3) P-CAS pathology total; (4) BCQ total; (5) YSR pathology total; (6) CAS pathology total; (7) CAFAS functioning; (8) GLOF.

[12]The four outcomes (numbered as in Tables 3.13–3.15) were: (9) presenting problem: parent-reported pathology; (10) parent-reported "most severe" pathology; (11) presenting problem: child-reported pathology; (12) child-reported "most severe" pathology.

Table 3.12. Summary of Significant Baseline Differences between Sites

		Child and family background		
Variable	Respondent	More "negative" site	$p(\alpha)^a$	ES^b
Demographics				
Socioeconomic status (education)	Primary caretaker	Comparison	<0.01	0.25
Military background				
Branch of service	Primary caretaker	NA	<0.01	NA
Deployment	Primary caretaker	Demonstration	0.03	NA
Prior system involvement				
Mental health service use	Primary caretaker	Comparison	<0.01	0.33
School attendance	Primary caretaker	Comparison	0.02	NA
Arrest	Primary caretaker	Comparison	<0.01	NA
		Mental health status of children		
Dysthymia	Primary caretaker	Comparison	0.01	0.16
Overanxious	Primary caretaker	Comparison	0.04	0.12
Posttraumatic stress disorder	Primary caretaker	Comparison	0.01	NA
Phobia				
Simple	Primary caretaker	Demonstration	0.05	NA
School	Primary caretaker	Demonstration	0.02	NA
Total diagnostic endorsements	Child	Comparison	0.04	0.16
Dysthymia	Child	Comparison	0.02	0.18
Attention-deficit	Child	Comparison	0.01	0.19
Major depression	Child	Comparison	0.02	0.19
Social problems	Child	Comparison	0.04	0.21
Phobia, social	Child	Demonstration	0.01	NA
Global functioning	Interviewer	Comparison	0.02	0.14
Role performance	Interviewer	Demonstration	0.03	0.14
Behavior toward others/self	Interviewer	Demonstration	0.02	0.16
		Family well-being		
Life events				
Stressors	Primary caretaker	Comparison	0.05	0.13
Resources				
Adequacy	Primary caretaker	Comparison	<0.01	0.23
Adaptation				
Coherence	Primary caretaker	Comparison	<0.01	0.37

[a]Based on χ^2 for nominal (categorical) variables or one-way ANOVA for continuous variables.
[b]Effect size is the difference between Demonstration and Comparison means expressed in SDs.

Table 3.13. Rate of Attrition for 12 Key Outcome Measures

Outcome measure	Wave 2[a]			Wave 3[a]		
	Demo	Comp	$p(\chi^2)^b$	Demo	Comp	$p(\chi^2)^b$
1. Overall outcome	25%	24%	0.96	42%	40%	0.60
2. CBCL pathology total	20%	14%	0.03	32%	25%	0.01
3. P-CAS pathology total	20%	21%	0.72	38%	36%	0.48
4. BCQ total	21%	19%	0.42	35%	29%	0.05
5. YSR pathology total[c]	27%	29%	0.62	42%	30%	0.01
6. CAS pathology total[d]	23%	30%	0.05	40%	41%	0.74
7. CAFAS functioning	20%	21%	0.72	38%	36%	0.48
8. GLOF	20%	22%	0.61	38%	36%	0.61
9. Presenting problem: parent-reported pathology	20%	21%	0.76	38%	36%	0.51
10. Parent-reported "most severe" pathology	21%	18%	0.41	35%	32%	0.31
11. Presenting problem: child-reported pathology	23%	30%	0.07	40%	42%	0.72
12. Child-reported "most severe" pathology	23%	29%	0.10	40%	38%	0.65

[a]At Wave 2, 84% of the Evaluation Sample contributed some diagnostic data; at Wave 3, 73%. Data loss in this table exceeds these rates since some of the combined variables are dependent on other variables. If, for example, P-CAS, CAFAS, or BCQ is missing, the overall outcome is, by definition, also missing.
[b]Based on χ^2 for nominal (categorical) variables.
[c]YSR for $N = 412$ with Wave 1 YSR. Children under 12 do not complete the YSR.
[d]CAS for $N = 675$ with Wave 1 CAS. Children under 8 do not complete the CAS.

the amount of missing data varied; (2) whether children whose cases had missing data differed clinically from children whose cases were not missing data; and (3) whether children whose cases had missing data had different outcomes.

Rates of Missing Data by Sites

The simplest test for biases in outcome appears in Table 3.13, which presents rates of missing data for the 12 mental health outcome measures discussed in Chapter 6. When the rate of data loss differs between sites, there is risk that outcome results are biased by differential attrition. Table 3.13 shows 24 results of tests for differences between the sites, expressed in rates of missing data. By chance, 5% of the results might be significant, so the Bonferroni correction for multiple significance was applied with an adjusted alpha level of $p < 0.002$. There were no site differences significant at $p < 0.002$.

Clinical Differences of Children Whose Cases Are Missing Data

A strong correlation between a methodological problem, such as attrition, and the topic of study, mental health outcome in two systems of care, could confound methodological difference with substantive outcome. We explored such relationships between missing data and mental health scores at Wave 1. If, for example, children with missing data had more serious mental health problems, the possibility of attrition[13] being confounded with mental health outcome[14] could not be ignored.

Table 3.14 reports 48 significance tests[15] of Wave 1 means by site and attrition. A main effect of attrition would mean that cases missing data at Wave 3, for example, had more serious psychopathology at Wave 1. A site-by-attrition interaction would mean that significant relationships between attrition and pathology differed[16] in the Demonstration and Comparison sites. By chance, 5% (2.4) of these tests might appear significant at the alpha level $p < 0.05$. A Bonferroni-corrected alpha level of $p < 0.001$ was applied. Three results significant at the 5% level were not significant at this adjusted level. These chance results revealed no clinical differences in children with missing data.

Outcome of Cases Missing Follow-Up Data

Indirect tests of possible outcome biases, such as the previous two, merely show that it is possible that "data dropouts" might influence mental health outcome in a statistically significant way. A few families

---

[13]"Attrition" in this analysis denotes a case with missing data at Wave 2 or Wave 3. Data loss could result because a participant either skipped a wave of data collection or participated but had missing data points.

[14]For example, if cases with missing data had severe mental health problems, then the site with the most attrition could appear to have superior outcome because cases with high pathology at Wave 1 tend to improve more than cases with milder pathology. While such a linkage may appear far-fetched, it cannot be dismissed a priori.

[15]General linear models (GLMs) in ANOVAs with models in the form Wave 1 = Site Attrition, where attrition (0, 1) means data missing at Wave 2 or Wave 3.

[16]For example, if attritors exhibited more psychopathology at the Demonstration site and less psychopathology at the Comparison site, then the interaction would be significant. Such an interaction could bias results. If sites were otherwise equal, the interaction would cause missing cases to push the site means in opposite directions.

Table 3.14. Score Biases in Attrition: Wave 1 versus Attrition

Outcome variable	Wave 2 $p(\alpha)^a$		Wave 3 $p(\alpha)^a$	
	Attrition	Site × Attrition	Attrition	Site × Attrition
1. Overall outcome	0.98	0.48	0.78	0.68
2. CBCL pathology total	0.78	0.62	0.75	0.61
3. P-CAS pathology total	0.59	0.98	0.61	0.79
4. BCQ total	0.85	0.11	0.53	0.28
5. YSR pathology total	0.43	0.64	0.06	0.50
6. CAS pathology total	0.14	0.31	0.51	0.38
7. CAFAS functioning competence	0.35	0.46	0.41	0.19
8. GLOF	0.25	0.39	0.21	0.78
9. Presenting problem: parent-reported pathology	0.58	0.94	0.98	0.72
10. Parent-reported "most severe" pathology	0.34	0.61	0.31	0.80
11. Presenting problem: child-reported pathology	0.08	0.22	0.04^b	0.93
12. Child-reported "most severe" pathology	0.02^b	0.09	0.04^b	0.20

^{a}Based on one-way ANOVA for continuous variables.
$^b p \leqslant 0.05$.

completely withdrew from the study. Much more frequently, families refused to participate in a given follow-up wave. Thus, there were many cases missing at Wave 3 who had data for Wave 2 and cases missing at Wave 2 who had data at Wave 3. By contrasting these partially missing cases against nonmissing cases, it was possible to detect whether "missingness" influenced outcome and whether that influence was similar for the Demonstration and Comparison sites. This analysis was done using a covariance analysis[17] much like that used in Chapter 6 to study site differences in mental health outcomes.

Table 3.15 presents the 12 key outcome measures at Wave 2 and Wave 3. The columns for Wave 2 outcome show the probability of the main effect "missingness"[18] and the probability of an interaction of "missingness" and site. These tests would be significant if there were large differences be-

[17]The GLMs were: [Wave 2 = (Site | Missing) Wave 1] and [Wave 3 = (Site | Missing) Wave 1]. In this case, missing refers to missing Wave 2 when the dependent variable is outcome at Wave 3. Wave 3 and Wave 1 refer to one of the 12 key dependent variables at Wave 1 (intake) or Wave 3 (outcome).
[18]Missing Wave 3.

Table 3.15. Probabilities for Site Differences in Outcome in Cases Missing Follow-Up

Outcome variable	Wave 2		Wave 3	
	$p(\alpha)^a$ (Wave 3 Missing)	$p(\alpha)^a$ (Missing W3 × Site)	$p(\alpha)^a$ (Wave 2 Missing)	$p(\alpha)^a$ (Missing W2 × Site)
1. Overall outcome	0.84	0.16	0.07	0.12
2. CBCL pathology total	0.80	0.70	0.69	0.53
3. P-CAS pathology total	0.36	0.40	0.03	0.73
4. BCQ total	0.86	0.61	0.07	0.04
5. YSR pathology total	0.94	0.59	0.69	0.20
6. CAS pathology total	0.69	0.38	0.00	0.19
7. CAFAS functioning competence[d]	0.99	0.26	0.05	0.04
8. GLOF[e]	0.05	0.07	0.32	0.35
9. Presenting problem: parent-reported pathology	0.61	0.82	0.02	0.98
10. Parent-reported "most severe" pathology	0.97	0.20	0.12	0.77
11. Presenting problem: child-reported pathology[f]	0.62	0.51	0.00	0.24
12. Child-reported "most severe" pathology[g]	0.90	0.50	0.03	0.47

[a] Based on one-way ANOVA for continuous variables.

[b] Children with nonmissing Wave 2 P-CAS have better outcome on Wave 3 P-CAS.

[c] Children with missing Wave 2 BCQ have slightly worse outcome on Wave 3 BCQ but only at the Comparison site ($p = 0.008$), not at the Demonstration site ($p = 0.85$).

[d] Children with missing Wave 2 CAFAS have more impairment at Wave 3. This difference occurs mainly at the Comparison site ($p = 0.006$), not the Demonstration site ($p = 0.96$).

[e] Children missing GLOF scores at Wave 3 have slightly less favorable outcome at Wave 2.

[f] Children missing Wave 2 "presenting problem" pathology scores report less favorable Wave 3 outcome on this variable.

[g] Children missing Wave 2 "most severe" pathology scores report less favorable Wave 3 outcome on this variable.

tween the Demonstration and Comparison sites in how "missingness" affected outcome.[19] Table 3.15 presents 48 significance tests, in which 8 differences are significant at the 5% level (6 main effects and 2 interactions). Of the 6 significant main effects, 5 revealed no bias, because the rates of attrition for these variables in Table 3.13 do not differ between sites for Wave 2 or Wave 3.[20] The 2 interactions do indicate a potential source of outcome bias, since the sites may differ in whether missing cases are higher or lower in psychopathology. However, both these interactions were barely significant ($p = 0.04$). Moreover, none of the findings met the Bonferroni-adjusted alpha level of $p < 0.001$. The outcomes for children whose cases were missing data did not differ from those for children whose cases were not missing data.

Summary of Attrition-Related Bias

Attrition was studied as a possible source of distortion of the results of the Outcome Study. At no point was there reason to conclude that differential attrition would affect outcomes.

REPRESENTATIVENESS OF THE EVALUATION SAMPLE

Generalizability of the findings of the Outcome Study depends on whether a continuum of care would work as well for other populations as for the families in the Evaluation Sample. This section compares the Evaluation Sample to other groups for whom comparable data were available:

- Military children who received mental health services in the *Project* catchment areas but were not part of the outcome Evaluation.
- Military children in *other* catchment areas receiving mental health services.
- Civilian children *in treatment*.

---

[19]An example of this interaction would be if missing cases had better outcome at one site and worse outcome at the other, or if missing cases had worse outcome at one site, but no difference at the other site.

[20]The 6 significant main effects (numbered as in Tables 3.13–3.15) were: (8) GLOF, (3) P-CAS pathology total, (6) CAS pathology total, (7) CAFAS functioning, (11) child-reported presenting problem, and (12) child-reported most severe pathology. The difference in the sites' rate of attrition was barely significant ($p = 0.05$) at Wave 2 for CAS pathology total only (Table 3.13).

The Evaluation Sample and Treated Population in the Catchment Area

Demographic and Military Profiles

Table 3.16 shows profiles of families in the Evaluation Sample and the nonevaluation groups in their respective catchment areas who received mental health treatment from October 1, 1991, through September 30, 1992.[21] Overall, at the Demonstration site, children in the Evaluation Sample were similar to their nonevaluation peers. However, the Evaluation Sample was younger and disproportionately from Air Force families. At the Comparison site, the two groups were rather similar, but the Evaluation Sample overrepresented males and children whose sponsor was enlisted military rather than an officer. Evaluation families with a member on active duty status were somewhat underrepresented at both sites. Overall, the Evaluation Sample's demographic characteristics appear similar to those of the total population of children treated at the Demonstration and Comparison sites.

Mental Health

At the outset, the Project intentionally oversampled children in more restrictive care. Because our primary research question focused on change in mental health status, representativeness of mental health profiles was of special interest. Table 3.17 shows the presenting diagnoses[22] given all children served at the Demonstration and Comparison sites, both in the Evaluation Sample and in the larger treated population. Overall, the Evaluation Sample was representative of the treated population at both the Demonstration site and the Comparison site. The same four diagnoses (attention-deficit, behavioral, mood, and adjustment disorders) described about 75% of the Evaluation Sample and nonevaluation groups at both sites. While there were a few statistically significant differences (four at the Demonstration site and three at the Comparison site), one at each site would be expected by chance alone. Moreover, none met the conservative Bonferroni-adjusted alpha of $p = 0.004$.

Additional measures of psychopathology were available to the Project

---

[21]A full year of data on the catchment area samples was available for fiscal year 1992. Fiscal year 1992 also overlaps with the recruitment phase of the Evaluation.

[22]These diagnoses were given by treating clinicians; they were not derived from the clinical interviews of the Project.

Table 3.16. Demographic and Military Profiles of Evaluation Sample and Treated Population in the Catchment Area

Characteristic	Demonstration site			Comparison site		
	Evaluation Sample	$p(\alpha)^a$	Treated population	Evaluation Sample	$p(\alpha)^a$	Treated population
Gender						
Male	62.0%	NS	59.9%	64.0%	0.02	57.7%
Female	38.0%		40.1%	36.0%		42.3%
Age						
5–7 years	26.4%	<0.01	12.5%	20.7%	NS	19.7%
8–11 years	26.1%		34.1%	25.1%		24.3%
12–17 years	47.5%		53.4%	54.2%		56.0%
Race						
White	72.0%	NS	67.3%	70.0%	—	NA
African-American	17.8%		21.8%	15.5%	—	NA
Other	10.2%		10.9%	14.5%	—	NA
Military status						
Active	78.3%	<0.01	83.6%	75.1%	0.02	79.9%
Nonactive	21.7%		16.4%	24.9%		20.1%
Rank						
Enlisted	84.5%	NS	83.2%	90.7%	<0.01	82.1%
Warrant officer	7.2%		9.9%	5.3%		8.7%
Officer	8.3%		6.9%	4.0%		9.2%
Branch						
Army	84.0%	0.02	88.6%	95.0%	NS	93.2%
Air Force	13.4%		9.8%	3.0%		3.7%
Navy	1.8%		0.8%	1.2%		2.6%
Marines	0.4%		0.3%	0.5%		0.5%
Other	0.4%		0.5%	0.3%		0.0%

^{a}Based on χ^2 for nominal (categorical) variables.

for children served at the Demonstration site,[23] for both the Evaluation and nonevaluation samples. Table 3.18 is based on standardized CBCL scores; the last three columns compare the Evaluation Sample with the non-evaluation sample. The proportion of children in the clinical ranges, as well as mean scores on syndrome and total scores, were significantly higher (more pathological) for the Evaluation Sample. These differences reflect the Project's intentional oversampling of children with more serious problems (i.e., those from inpatient and residential settings). Table 3.18 also

[23]The Rumbaugh Management Information System (MIS) contained these sample data. Similar comparisons could not be made for the Comparison site.

Table 3.17. Presenting Diagnoses of Evaluation and Nonevaluation Children

| | Demonstration site | | | | | | Comparison site | | | | | |
| | Evaluation Sample | | Treated population[a] | | | Evaluation Sample | | Treated population[a] | | |
Diagnosis	N	%	N	%	$p(\chi^2)^b$	N	%	N	%	$p(\chi^2)^b$
Anxiety disorder	22	3.9	322	5.9	NS	9	4.0	176	6.9	NS
Attention-deficit disorder	77	13.8	1013	18.6	0.05	40	18.0	564	22.1	NS
Behavioral disorders	127	22.8	1079	19.8	NS	40	18.0	280	10.9	0.01
Eating disorders	2	0.4	17	0.3	NS	2	1.0	8	0.3	NS
Mood disorder/depression	104	18.7	928	17.0	NS	48	21.6	338	13.2	0.01
Adjustment disorder	89	16.0	1097	20.1	0.05	49	22.1	658	25.7	NS
Psychoses	5	0.9	55	1.0	NS	5	2.2	46	1.8	NS
Substance-related	32	5.8	142	2.6	0.01	3	1.4	56	2.2	NS
Physiological	28	5.0	236	4.3	NS	0	—	92	3.6	0.01
Personality disorder	15	2.7	71	1.3	0.05	1	0.4	12	0.5	NS
Delayed development	52	9.3	461	8.4	NS	2	0.9	79	3.1	NS
Other	4	0.7	40	0.7	NS	23	10.4	249	9.7	NS
TOTALS	557	100	5461	100		222	100	2558	100	

[a]Data for the treated population are from the MIS and CHAMPUS files for the Demonstration and Comparison sites, respectively, and represent all cases throughout the Demonstration period. Treated population totals do not include participants in the Evaluation Sample.
[b]Significance based on 2 × 2 cell (1) for each diagnosis within the overall 12 × 2 diagnosis by sample crosstabulation.

Table 3.18. Psychopathology Measures for Evaluation and Nonevaluation Children at the Demonstration Site[a]

Variable	Inpatient/RTC (N = 37)	More than outpatient (N = 131)	Outpatient (N = 404)	Evaluation Sample (N = 574)	Nonevaluation (N = 2220)	p(α)[b]
Clinical						
Competence	48%	63%	49%	52%	29%	<0.01
Problems	77%	77%	57%	63%	52%	<0.01
Internalizing	51%	62%	43%	47%	40%	0.01
Externalizing	77%	84%	48%	58%	46%	<0.01
Internalizing or externalizing	86%	90%	64%	71%	59%	<0.01
Total competence	36	34	39	38	41	<0.01
Total problems	67	70	64	65	63	<0.01
Internalizing	64	66	61	62	60	<0.01
Externalizing	67	71	63	65	62	<0.01
Withdrawn	64	66	61	62	60	<0.01
Somatic	61	61	59	59	58	0.03
Anxious/depressed	64	66	62	63	61	<0.01
Social problems	58	63	60	61	60	0.01
Thought disorders	64	66	61	62	61	<0.01
Attention problems	62	67	65	65	63	<0.01
Delinquency	67	71	63	65	62	<0.01
Aggressiveness	66	70	64	65	63	<0.01
Sex problems	61	55	55	55	54	0.12

[a]Data are based on Achenbach's CBCL, administered at the Rumbaugh Clinic to all clients, and by the Evaluation Sample to all study participants. Evaluation Sample CBCL data were used when the Rumbaugh data were missing for Evaluation cases. Correlations between Evaluation Sample means and treated population means ranged from 0.44 to 0.73 for global measures and Syndrome Scales. Only two correlations were lower than 0.60, and all were significant. Level of care information was missing for two cases; they are excluded from that analysis.
[b]Based on χ² for nominal (categorical) variables or one-way ANOVA for continuous variables.

Table 3.19. Profiles of the Evaluation Sample
and Other Military Children in Treatment[a]

Characteristic	Evaluation Sample[b]	Other military samples[c]
Demographic		
Mean age	11.1	11.9
Male	63%	59%
Military		
Enlisted	87%	94%
Officer	13%	6%
Psychopathology		
Psychosis	1%	4%
Schizophrenia	1%	1%
Hyperactivity	28%	31%
Drug abuse	0	1%
Alcoholism	16%	2%
No diagnosis	3%	2–4%

[a]Psychometric information or information concerning methods employed by other
studies was insufficient to conduct statistical tests of differences between the two
groups.
[b]In the Evaluation Sample, psychosis and schizophrenia are measured by the same
variable (see Chapter 2).
[c]In other military samples, Morrison (1981) reports on schizophrenia and LaGrone
(1978) reports on psychosis. Also, Morrison reports 2% of his sample with no
diagnosis; LaGrone, 4%.

shows that when only the most commonly utilized level of care, outpatient
treatment, is considered, the Demonstration's Evaluation and nonevaluation samples were similar.[24]

The Evaluation Sample and Other Military Children
Receiving Services

Table 3.19 compares the Evaluation Sample with other samples of
clinic-referred military children reported by Morrison (1981) and LaGrone
(1978). Demographically, the Evaluation sample was very similar to these
other samples. However, a higher proportion of Evaluation Sample
CHAMPUS sponsors (13%) were officers than those reported in the other
two studies. Data on psychopathology were limited for these comparisons,
both in the number of diagnostic categories reported and because of the
dissimilar methods by which measures were obtained. Nonetheless, the

[24]At the time of entry into the study, 71% of the Evaluation Sample were receiving outpatient
services.

distribution of disorders was similar for the two groups, with the notewor-thy exceptions of alcoholism and psychosis. Both groups, however, had nearly the same proportion of children for whom no clinical diagnosis was warranted.

As discussed in Chapter 1, the Demonstration and the Evaluation Project were designed to explore the effectiveness of a continuum-of-care model for delivering mental health services to military families. The possi-bility of replicating this model in other military communities is therefore of interest. The information thus far presented indicates that the children in the Evaluation Sample were not unlike other military dependents in treat-ment, either in the Project catchment areas or the larger military popula-tion. Thus, the findings presented in Chapter 6 may generalize to other military settings.

The Evaluation Sample and Civilian Children in Treatment

In this time of debate over health care reform, and in the absence of other studies, the results of the Evaluation should be of interest with regard to civilian populations of youth. A potential threat to the gener-alizability of the findings is the fact that all children in the Evaluation had some past or current affiliation with the military. LaGrone (1978) has identified a "military family syndrome" characterized by authoritarian fathers, depressed mothers, and behaviorally disordered children. Recent empirical data show, however, that psychological profiles of military wives are similar to those of their civilian counterparts (Fernandez-Pol, 1988), frequent relocation is unrelated to increased emotional or behavioral problems among military spouses or children (Marchant & Medway, 1987), and father's absence under routine conditions has no adverse effects on the psychological well-being of military spouses and children (Jensen, Grogan, Xenakis, & Bain, 1989). Further, the prevalence of conduct dis-order and other disorders is similar in referred (Morrison, 1981) and non-referred (Jensen et al., 1991) populations of civilian and military children. These data suggest that the military status of the Evaluation Sample does not preclude the applicability of Project findings for civilian youth with mental health needs.

Table 3.20 presents the mean CBCL and YSR scores for the Evaluation Sample and the range of mean scores reported for civilian children re-ferred for treatment (Achenbach, 1991).[25] The third column shows the

---

[25]Achenbach's ranges are based on the lowest and highest mean he reports for each gender and age group on each variable. His description of the civilian samples suggests that they are fairly representative of the total United States population.

Table 3.20. Clinical Profiles of the Evaluation Sample
and Civilian Children Referred for Treatment

Mean scale scores[a]	Evaluation Sample	Referred civilians	Range of differences
CBCL			
Total competence	36.0	37.7–39.8	−1.7 to −3.8
Total problems	65.2	63.8–64.4	+1.4 to +0.8
Total externalizing	64.2	61.2–62.8	+3.0 to +1.4
Total internalizing	62.3	61.4–62.0	+0.9 to +0.3
YSR			
Total competence	40.0	43.6–44.8	−3.6 to −4.8
Total problems	58.6	58.0–60.5	+0.6 to −1.9
Total externalizing	59.9	56.8–59.8	+3.1 to +0.1
Total internalizing	56.5	56.9–59.3	−0.4 to −2.8

[a]Mean scale scores are standardized T-scores.

difference between the mean scores for the Evaluation and civilian samples. Most differences are quite small. Moreover, some means of the Evaluation Sample are higher and others are lower than those for the civilian youth. The general similarity between the Evaluation and civilian samples suggests that the Outcome Study findings may be generalizable to non-military populations of children in treatment.

SUMMARY

This chapter described the Evaluation Sample in terms of the comparability of families and children at the Demonstration and Comparison sites at the time the Project began. Site differences in data loss during the course of the Evaluation were also examined. Further, the sample's representativeness of other children—military and civilian—in treatment was considered. Baseline comparisons showed that the sites were very similar on a wide range of variables salient for assessing mental health outcomes. Moreover, sites did not vary appreciably with regard to the amount of data or the types of cases available for the outcome analyses. These findings help to dispel worries associated with the lack of random assignment and differential attrition. Finally, the data suggested that the Evaluation Sample was similar in many ways to other groups of children in treatment. Thus, the continuum of care implemented at the Demonstration site could be expected to have similar outcomes for other children with mental health needs.

4

Access and the Intake and Assessment Process

This chapter addresses the program operations and outcomes of the intake and assessment process at the Demonstration and Comparison sites. The intake and assessment process is an integral part of the continuum-of-care concept. Figure 1.1 is reproduced here as Figure 4.1 to illustrate the conceptual framework of how intake and assessment fit into the program model being tested. In a continuum-of-care approach, the needs of the child determine service delivery instead of service availability determining treatment. This approach requires a thorough and accurate assessment of the child's needs at intake. The use of a standardized and coordinated intake and assessment process was recently advocated by the Practice Directorate of the American Psychological Association (1992) in their response to growing public concern over managed care. Their *integrated care* strategy draws on the principle that it makes sense to "get it right the first time." Unlike most approaches to managed care, integrated care encourages companies to make use of high-quality providers at the "front end" of the treatment process, placing special emphasis on careful psychological assessment at intake.

The following section describes the intake and assessment processes at the Demonstration and Comparison sites. The effects of these processes on ratings of adequacy and quality by community experts are also discussed. The characteristics of the treated population and their utilization of intake and assessment services are reviewed in the second section. Finally, consumer views of and their satisfaction with the intake and assessment procedures at the Demonstration and Comparison sites are presented in the third section.

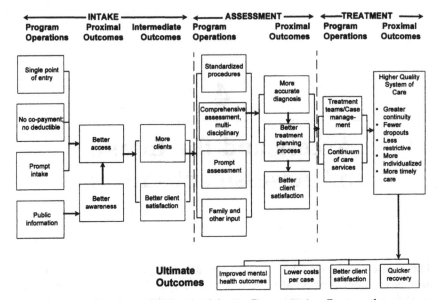

Figure 4.1. Fort Bragg Child and Adolescent Demonstration: Program theory.

DESCRIPTION OF THE INTAKE AND ASSESSMENT PROCESS

Intake and Assessment at the Demonstration Site

One important feature of the Demonstration model was a single point of entry into the continuum of care, allowing for a central, standardized, and coordinated intake process. The overriding purpose of intake and assessment at the Demonstration site was

> to ensure that clients' needs will be responded to in a timely and consistent manner

in accordance with a policy

> to assure that clients who meet criteria for admission to Rumbaugh Clinic services will be responded to in an appropriate manner that promotes continuity of care (Cardinal Mental Health Group, 1990a).

Generally, procedures stipulated that all potential clients who initially called or walked in be screened for both clinical and Civilian Health and Medical Program of the Uniformed Services (CHAMPUS) eligibility. The location of the contact was not always the Rumbaugh Clinic; however, uniform procedures and admission criteria governed the process. If the child was not eligible, indicated referrals were made and the screening form was placed in an ineligible file. If the child met criteria for admission, a determination was made about the urgency of his or her problem (i.e., medical emergency, psychiatric emergency, priority or routine intake). Intake and assessment was to be completed within 2 hours of initial contact for medical or psychiatric emergency cases and within 7 days for priority cases. For routine cases, intakes were to be scheduled within 21 days.

Emergency intake and assessment usually consisted of crisis intervention and crisis management. Intake staff were on emergency call during business hours for a 1-week period every 6 weeks. Intake clinicians had no other responsibilities during their emergency on-call week. After-hours emergencies were managed by Rumbaugh Clinic staff (who received additional monetary compensation) on a voluntary basis. For routine intake and assessment, the child and the child's parent(s) or guardian(s) (hereinafter referred to as "parent") arrived 30 minutes before the scheduled intake appointment to complete any necessary paperwork. At the time of the appointment, the intake clinician met with both the child and the parent to discuss confidentiality and choices in treatment providers and to obtain consent to release information. The clinician then interviewed the child and parent individually, using a standardized interview and form. The parent also completed several questionnaires regarding the child's developmental history and family situation. Before the child and parent left the Clinic, the clinician reviewed the questionnaires for completeness.

With the interviews over, the clinician completed a measure of the child's psychosocial functioning. Staff members then met to review the child's case within 2 working days of the intake and assessment. This meeting was led by a child psychiatrist or psychologist with the intake clinician, case manager, and other relevant staff members in attendance. Once the child was accepted as a client, parents were considered part of the treatment team and invited to participate in subsequent treatment meetings. They were not included, however, in this initial intake staff meeting, which focused on the establishment of a preliminary treatment plan.

The need for further psychological or medical assessment was determined on a case-by-case basis at the intake staff meeting. The child's case was then assigned to the most appropriate level of treatment. In the overwhelming majority of cases, this meant referral to an outpatient therapist in the community who was under contract to the Demonstration. However, the decision could include any level of care if the indicated criteria were met.

The diagnostic criteria for initial eligibility and the functioning criteria that determined level of initial care were viewed as "gatekeeping" mechanisms and were subjected to many layers of monitoring, both internally and externally. The standardized intake process and intake staff meeting provided a more comprehensive and structured approach than is required through CHAMPUS and, indeed, exceeded most of the procedures used in the mental health field according to expert reviewers (Bickman et al., 1993; Haberkern, 1991; Phillips & Edwards, 1993).

The intake clinician was responsible for crisis intervention and referral prior to the initial staff meeting. The case was to be staffed in less than 2 days if deemed emergency or priority. In these instances, a clinical case manager or outpatient therapist was assigned the case and was responsible to contact the parent to arrange treatment.

Additionally, the Demonstration had a "no reject" requirement:

> Children often tend to be excluded, expelled from, or refused entry to programs because they are very difficult to serve, have multiple problems, do not fit the established program "model," are defined as "untreatable," or do not otherwise meet established program criteria. The obligation of our program is to accept responsibility for treatment of emotionally disturbed children and to revise and adjust services using innovative approaches when appropriate (Cardinal Mental Health Group, 1990b).

These children are often unserved or "fall through the cracks" between multiple providers in the service system; the Demonstration, through its cost reimbursement contract and in contrast to many disincentives existing in other settings, was able to admit and serve these children.

Intake and Assessment at the Comparison Site

At the Comparison site, neither a single point of entry nor a standardized intake and assessment procedure was uniformly in place. In traditional CHAMPUS treatment, a child's parent contacts an eligible service provider, who then decides whether the child is appropriate for treatment. Eligibility criteria and intake procedures vary by provider; timelines for intake are typically determined by the provider's caseload. The range of service providers includes outpatient therapists, inpatient hospitals, and residential treatment centers (RTCs).

Even though the Army contract with the state of North Carolina specifically stated that no other demonstration projects were to be allowed to affect the Demonstration and Evaluation Projects, changes affecting CHAMPUS benefits have taken place and influenced the manner in which families accessed their benefits at the Comparison site. In October 1990, the total annual benefits for outpatient, inpatient, and residential treatment were reduced. Of even greater impact was the implementation of a procedure for precertification of all admissions to hospitals and RTCs by a contracted managed care company, Health Management Strategies International, Inc. (HMS). Such admissions had been previously approved by signature of an admitting physician; after October 1990, a preadmission review by HMS was required. Children who would typically have been admitted to a hospital or an RTC for an extended period were being denied CHAMPUS coverage in many cases. Not only did this procedure limit the number of admissions, but also, when approval was given, it was for shorter preapproved lengths of treatment.

In addition, the Army managed-care initiative entitled Gateway to Care was implemented at both Comparison site locations during the course of the Project. Gateway was formally adopted at Fort Campbell for fiscal year 1992 (starting October 1991) and at Fort Stewart for fiscal year 1993. As part of Gateway, a number of mechanisms were used to encourage CHAMPUS beneficiaries to access mental health care through the local post hospital instead of going directly to community CHAMPUS providers. The ultimate goal of Gateway was to control both hospital and CHAMPUS mental health expenditures.

Under a fully implemented Gateway model, all mental health services would be accessed by referral from the primary care clinic on post. During the period examined by the Evaluation, however, only partial implementation had taken place. At both Fort Campbell and Fort Stewart, inpatient, residential, and outpatient mental health care were available through CHAMPUS via the mechanisms described below.

Psychiatric Hospital Admissions

Psychiatric hospital admissions, as the most expensive type of care, were highlighted for intensive review under Gateway. All inpatient psychiatric admissions were screened for approval on post. For admission, a Nonavailability of Services (NAS) form had to be approved by the hospital's commander or designee (at the Comparison site, the Department of Psychiatry) and entered into the Defense Enrollment Eligibility Reporting System (DEERS) computer base. HMS would consider precertification only if the NAS was in the DEERS system; then, HMS conducted an additional precertification process as discussed above.

Length of stay, or payment therefore, was handled by HMS through its ongoing certification process. HMS usually precertified only a few days for diagnostic and evaluation purposes; the hospital then had to obtain approval for extended treatment. HMS informed the local Army post hospital's coordinated care division of all admissions.

Gateway implementation plans at both Fort Campbell and Fort Stewart called for reduction in inpatient utilization. At Fort Campbell, the initial focus was on children; at Fort Stewart, it was primarily on adults. At both sites, any referral for inpatient care was scrutinized on post before an NAS form was issued and delivery of psychiatric inpatient treatment on post had been either planned or implemented.

Residential Treatment Center Admissions

RTC admissions were governed by rules separate from those for hospitalization and did not procedurally require on-post screening and approval through the NAS process. HMS did, however, precertify these admissions similarly to inpatient stays, with the exception that it did not require the NAS form to be in the DEERS system first. Again, payment for length of stay was determined by HMS. HMS informed the local post hospital's coordinated care division of all precertified CHAMPUS admissions in its catchment area.

It should be noted that Fort Campbell, using NAS forms (not complying with CHAMPUS procedures), implemented on-post review and approval of RTC admissions during early fiscal year 1992. As discussed in Chapter 7, this procedure appeared to significantly reduce admissions. Review of Fort Campbell procedures later by the Inspector General of the Army required that they follow standard procedures.

Outpatient Admissions

Outpatient services did not require any on-post screening or approval in order to be paid by CHAMPUS if both provider and client were eligible. HMS precertified services only for intensive (more than two sessions per week) or long-term (more than 23 visits in 1 year) outpatient therapy.

At both Comparison site locations, however, extensive marketing was directed to CHAMPUS beneficiaries and community CHAMPUS providers to encourage (or provide the perception that it was required to participate in) a review by the post hospital's psychiatry clinic. At both sites, efforts were made to provide more outpatient services to children (at no cost) through the psychiatry clinic and other on-post services. Knowledge of these services appeared to increase on-post contacts. Fort Campbell instituted a "disengagement" form to show that a child who had been screened by the psychiatry clinic and found eligible for services that could not be served on post was being referred to a CHAMPUS provider in the community.

Other Intake Issues

Through Gateway, some mechanisms were put into place to screen admissions to all treatment settings. However, several aspects of the continuum of care available at the Demonstration site were missing at the Comparison site. First, no uniform policy or procedures existed regarding who was eligible for services or how access to services was to be handled. Second, no standardized screening or admission process was put into place within or across service settings. Third, in the cost-containment environment of Army hospitals during this period, there were strong incentives to deny the use of inpatient or residential care. Furthermore, cost shifting of difficult-to-treat children to the public sector was encouraged. For instance, Gateway implementation at Fort Campbell coincided with the expansion of the range of services available to children in the custody of the State of Tennessee (Maloy, 1994). Parents of children who would previously have been served in inpatient or residential treatment settings using their CHAMPUS benefits were instructed to place their children in State custody for such services. Since the Project was designed to capture the service use of those children who actually used their CHAMPUS benefits, it was not possible to evaluate such CHAMPUS-eligible children who did not use their benefits.

Summary

The intake and assessment process is an integral part of the continuum-of-care concept. One important feature of the Demonstration site was a single point of entry into the continuum of care, allowing for a central, standardized, and coordinated intake process. The Demonstration implemented a single point of entry with both fidelity to its proposed model and high quality (Bickman et al., 1993; Heflinger, 1993). In contrast, at the Comparison site, neither a single point of entry nor a standardized intake and assessment procedure was uniformly in place. The effects of these differing methods of accessing child mental health care are discussed below in relation to ratings by community experts, utilization patterns, and reports of satisfaction with services.

Ratings by Community Experts

As part of the Implementation Study (Heflinger, 1993), community experts in the Project catchment areas responded to a written survey assessing adequacy, quality, and service system performance of the mental health system for military dependents in those communities. As shown in Table 4.1, these community experts, including psychologists, psychiatrists, social workers, school and juvenile court personnel, and Army personnel, rated adequacy and quality of the intake and assessment process at the Demonstration site as significantly greater than at the Comparison site. In

Table 4.1. Community Ratings on Intake for Military Dependent Children[a]

Dimensions of intake and assessment	Demonstration site			Comparison site			ES	$p(t)$[b]
	Mean	SD	N	Mean	SD	N		
Adequacy of centralized intake	4.36[c]	0.75	44	2.54	1.28	54	1.75	<0.01
Quality of centralized intake	4.43[c]	0.76	44	2.70	1.22	40	1.77	<0.01
Service performance on access								
Making children and their families feel welcome and at ease in service settings	4.34[c]	0.75	38	3.28	1.00	46	1.19	<0.01
Preventing providers from treating only the easiest child clients and leaving difficult clients underserved and at risk	4.33[c]	0.84	39	2.89	1.09	53	1.50	<0.01
Making appropriate mental health services available to all children and families who need them	4.27[c]	0.86	45	2.75	1.13	67	1.50	<0.01
Preventing children from having to enter State custody to receive services	4.13[c]	0.92	39	2.72	1.11	50	1.38	<0.01
Avoiding excessive waiting lists or long delays in scheduling appointments	4.05[c]	0.91	44	2.30	1.02	57	1.80	<0.01
Offering services during evening and weekend hours	3.92[c]	0.98	37	2.35	1.03	54	1.60	<0.01
Placing services in locations easily accessible to families	3.88[c]	0.87	41	2.67	0.71	51	1.60	<0.01
Keeping "red tape" at a minimum in enrolling children in services	3.60[c]	1.25	42	2.45	1.10	51	0.98	<0.01

[a] Scale: 1 ("very poor") to 5 ("very good").
[b] From t-test between means.
[c] Significantly better performance at the Demonstration site than at the Comparison site at $p \leq 0.01$.

addition, on items assessing access to mental health care, they rated the Demonstration site significantly more positively. These differences were statistically significant with a large effect size (> 1 SD).

INTAKE AND ASSESSMENT UTILIZATION

The examination of utilization patterns of intake and assessment is another important aspect of understanding the Demonstration. This section describes the use of the specialized intake and assessment component at the Demonstration site and, when dimensions of the intake process were present at both sites, compares its services to those provided at the Comparison site. These dimensions include examination of access to services; single point of entry; community awareness; use of intake and assessment; utilization characterized as "one-visit-only"; timeliness of screenings, intake and assessment, treatment team meetings, and follow-up services; use of formal evaluation services and other facets of intake and assessment; treatment planning; and accuracy of diagnosis. These discussions complement the findings of the quality of intake and assessment presented in the Final Report of the Quality Study of the Fort Bragg Evaluation Project (Bickman et al., 1993, pp. 9–28).

Increased Access to Services

Measuring and comparing access to services was straightforward: In a simple comparison of two matched sites, the presumption is that the level of need is similar, and differences in utilization therefore reflect differences in access (Ruiz, 1993; Weisner & Schmidt, 1992). The measure of access used was the number of children served. To account for any differences in the size of the population of eligible clients, the percentage of eligible children served was examined as well (Coulam et al., 1990; Taube & Rupp, 1986). Two different methods of studying access to services were informative. The first comparison involved examining the catchment area surrounding Fort Bragg both before and after the start of the Demonstration. This examination was possible because CHAMPUS data were available for the Fort Bragg catchment area for fiscal years 1988 and 1989. The second comparison involved differences between the Demonstration and Comparison sites. Over time, both sites changed (i.e., the Demonstration matured as the program became operational and the "care as usual" system at the Comparison site continued to evolve). Thus, differences between the Demonstration and Comparison sites unfolded over time. Between-site comparisons were made both by fiscal year and then by

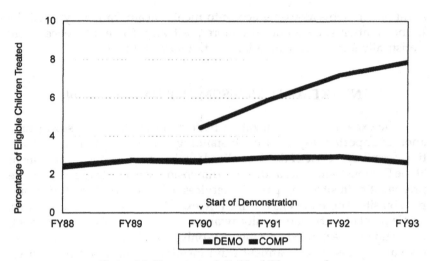

Figure 4.2. Percentage of eligible children served.

using combined data for fiscal years 1991, 1992, and 1993 (hereinafter referred to as the "Demonstration period").[1]

As shown in Figure 4.2, access at the Demonstration and Comparison sites was similar in each fiscal year prior to the Demonstration. Between 2% and 3% of eligible children received services. Since the catchment areas were of similar sizes, these percentages represented virtually identical numbers of children served (see Table 4.2). In fiscal year 1988, 938 children were served in the Fort Bragg catchment area; at the Comparison site, 949.

Table 4.2 and Figure 4.2 both show that the effect of the Demonstration on access was profound. The percentage of children served in each fiscal year during the Demonstration period was more than double that for fiscal years preceding the Demonstration (i.e., fiscal years 1988 and 1989) at either site. In addition, the Demonstration served more than twice as many

[1]Fiscal year 1990 was excluded from the Demonstration period because it is best viewed as a transition period. Data for the Demonstration period are based on records of individuals being served over a 3-year period; they are not a simple average of the figures for each year. Data for fiscal years do not control for duplication across years. For example, it is possible that a clinic may report having served 1000 clients per fiscal year for two consecutive fiscal years. However, if one examines those two fiscal years combined, it is not acceptable to assume that the number served was 2000. It may have been the case that only 1750 were served during that combined period because some clients could have been served in both fiscal years.

Table 4.2. Access: Number of Children Served
and Percentage of Eligible Children Served

	Demonstration		Comparison	
Time span	N	%	N	%
Fiscal year[a]				
1988	938	2.5%	949	2.4%
1989	1124	2.7%	1189	2.7%
1991	2648	6.0%	1322	2.9%
1992	3327	7.2%	1108	2.9%
1993	3572	8.0%	1145	2.7%
Demonstration period	6033	13.6%	2869	6.8%

[a]Fiscal year 1990 was omitted because the Demonstration was operational for only 4 months of that fiscal year. Fiscal year 1990 is best seen as a transition.

children as the Comparison site in each fiscal year following Demonstration start-up. During the Demonstration period, over 6000 children were served by the Demonstration. This number represents 13.6% of children who lived in the catchment area.[2] In contrast, the percentage of eligible children served at the Comparison site was 6.8%.

Access at the Demonstration site increased throughout the Demonstration period. During fiscal year 1993, 8% of children in the catchment area received mental health services through the Demonstration. Assuming that the current estimates of the need for mental health services among all children mentioned in Chapter 1 are correct, this increase brought children with a genuine need for treatment into the system. It is difficult to pinpoint the cause of the increased number of children in services; it may have been the result of eliminating cost-sharing by families, improving available services, enhancing community awareness, or increasing information available to parents. Regardless, at the most basic level, the Demonstration dramatically increased access to the service system.

[2]The 13.6% figure is not a measure of prevalence, but the number of children served divided by the average population of eligible children in the catchment area. Dividing by the average size served as a means of standardizing the measure for differences in catchment area size. A measure of prevalence, however, would use as a denominator the number of children who lived in the catchment area throughout the Demonstration period. Because families moved in and out of the catchment area during the Demonstration, this figure is no doubt larger than that of the number of children living in the catchment area on a specific date in a given year. A measure of the prevalence of mental health services use, therefore, would likely be less than 13.6%.

Single Point of Entry

The intake and assessment process at the Demonstration site was an outgrowth of the continuum-of-care treatment paradigm, which is based on an explicit set of assumptions about how to treat individual clients and how children should enter the mental health system. Each component was constructed to represent a particular element of the model so that an ideal standard would be implicit in the treatment system. Besides comparisons to the usual system of services, an important part of the evaluative process was to determine the extent to which the program (as implemented) corresponded to an ideal system of care. The Evaluation team investigated inconsistencies with the program model, as illustrated in Figure 4.1.

Important facets of the continuum of care include elimination of barriers to and the coordination of service through the establishment of a single point of entry to the mental health system. However, the single point of entry was not completely executed at the Demonstration site. The CHAMPUS contract with the fiscal intermediary for the Fort Bragg catchment area, Blue Cross/Blue Shield of South Carolina, did not require the fiscal intermediary to disallow claims for services covered by the Demonstration; thus, it was possible for claims submitted by local providers to be paid contrary to the design of the Demonstration. From October 1990 to September 1993, 1156 children were served through the CHAMPUS system in the Fort Bragg catchment area. The majority of services delivered to this group were low-cost (e.g., outpatient treatment), and 96% of the children received outpatient therapy as their most restrictive level of treatment. Almost half these children (526 of 1156) received services through both CHAMPUS and the Demonstration Project. However, 14% of the cases (166 of 1156) initially received CHAMPUS services and received all subsequent services from the Demonstration. Hence, the remaining 31% (360 of 1156) received services from both systems simultaneously. Although the Demonstration was successful in maintaining a single point of entry for those clients who received services through the Rumbaugh Clinic, it had little control over those who were able to access services through the traditional CHAMPUS system. The failure in the single point of entry was not the responsibility of the Demonstration, but the result of lack of a reimbursement policy between the Army and the fiscal intermediary.

Community Awareness

Data from the Final Report of the Implementation Study of the Fort Bragg Evaluation Project (Heflinger, 1993) addressed the extent to which the community was aware of the services available at the Demonstration site and the means by which to access those services. Representatives from community agencies, private practices, and the Army posts at the Demonstration and Comparison sites were polled in a network analysis and were asked to rate problems encountered by those seeking services. Of particular interest were area providers' and families' knowledge of and access to mental health services (see Table 4.1). There was a significant ($p < 0.01$) difference between the sites, indicating that both providers and families in the catchment area of the Demonstration were more aware of the availability of services and the means by which to access them. Another comparison made in the Implementation Study involved ratings of community awareness before and after the implementation of the Demonstration. Before the implementation of the Demonstration, 85% of the experts polled in the Demonstration catchment area rated awareness as a considerable problem, while the rate for the Comparison site was 64%. After Demonstration implementation, only 19% of the experts in the Demonstration area felt that the community's lack of awareness was a considerable problem, while 50% of experts felt it to be a problem at the Comparison site. Hence, according to ratings by experts, community awareness of mental health services, and the means by which to access them, increased dramatically with the implementation of the Demonstration.

Use of Intake and Assessment

In most cases, children entering the Demonstration were screened by telephone to appraise their clinical condition and to determine eligibility for treatment. As described above, the primary form of initial face-to-face contact was the intake and assessment. The intake and assessment process resulted in an intake staff meeting that served to develop an initial treatment plan. As was shown in Table 4.2, between October 1990 and September 1993, over 6000 clients received at least one service through the Demonstration. Of those clients served, 95.8% received formal intake and assessment, and for 88.4% a formal intake staff meeting was documented. Fewer than 4% of those served received more than one intake and assessment. The number and frequency of formal intake–assessments at the Comparison site is difficult to determine, since CHAMPUS claims used the same code for intake–assessment and individual therapy, although it is likely that the first several sessions of contact with each mental health provider were devoted to intake. While the Demonstration site used standardized intake procedures, however, intakes by mental health providers at the Comparison site were neither standardized nor coordinated. Thus, if a child received services from more than one provider, it was highly probable that multiple intake–assessments were performed.

Utilization Characterized as "One-Visit-Only"

At the Demonstration site, individuals who received an intake and assessment but no other services provided an important index of the quality of the intake and assessment process. Receiving only an intake and assessment but no further services may indicate a lower-quality process, given that it is unlikely that a single session would result in the resolution of a significant problem. The Comparison analog to this group would be those individuals who received only one outpatient visit. This analog assumes that in the traditional CHAMPUS system, initial visits served as intake and assessment. At the Demonstration site, only 7% of those served received only an intake and assessment and no further services. At the Comparison site, however, this was true for 24% of children served. Thus, over 3 times the number of children dropped out of care at the Comparison site after only one contact with a mental health professional. This result clearly illustrates the Demonstration's superiority to engage families and children in the treatment process.

Timeliness

Another important aspect of the continuum-of-care philosophy at the Demonstration site was that intake and assessment should proceed in a timely manner. The timeliness of this assessment would facilitate the process of forming and implementing an individualized treatment plan. The average lag time between the initial screening and the intake and assessment was 9 calendar days at the Demonstration site.

At the Demonstration site, the intake and assessment process took an average of 1.5 hours to complete. Once the intake and assessment was completed, an average of 3 calendar days passed before an intake staff meeting was convened. Upon development of the initial treatment plan, an average of another 14 calendar days passed before delivery of the first therapeutic service. This represents an average of 17 calendar days between intake and assessment and the receipt of the first therapeutic service.

For the purpose of between-site comparison, the initial outpatient visit at the Comparison site was used as the analog of the Demonstration's intake and assessment. An average of 38 calendar days passed between the initial visit and the first therapeutic service at the Comparison site, more than twice the lag time at the Demonstration site. These results confirmed perceptions of parents, adolescents, staff, and contractual providers (see Bickman et al., 1993; Heflinger, 1993) that Evaluation Sample participants at the Demonstration site were more satisfied with the timeliness and convenience of intake and assessment than those at the Comparison site. Consumer satisfaction with the intake and assessment process is discussed in depth below.

Use of Formal Evaluation Services and Other Facets of Intake and Assessment

Although the Comparison site did not use the same intake and assessment process as the Demonstration site, it nevertheless evaluated children's mental health status and need. One component of the evaluation process common to both the Demonstration and Comparison sites was the use of formal evaluations (e.g., intelligence tests, neuropsychological examinations, and specialized assessments). For both sites, then, it was possible to make comparisons regarding the relative use of formal evaluation procedures. According to utilization data for the treated population, 15% of the children served at the Demonstration site received a formal evaluation, whereas 56% of Comparison site clients received these services. The lower use of formalized assessment at the Demonstration site may have been a function of the quality of the intake–assessments being conducted. Contractual providers involved in the Demonstration Project felt that the Demonstration's intake–assessments were comprehensive and useful. Another explanation of the lower use of formalized assessment may be, however, that children at the Demonstration site were referred for additional formal psychological or medical testing only when indicated, whereas such referral occurred on a more routine basis at the Comparison site.

Parent reports also described differences in service experiences during the intake and assessment process at the Demonstration and Comparison sites, as can be seen in Table 4.3. Parents and children participated in interviews as part of the intake process more often at the Demonstration site. However, as noted above, more formal testing was performed during the intake process at the Comparison site. Approximately half of parents at each site reported that a treatment plan was developed for their child during the intake process, with more parents being directly involved in treatment planning at the Demonstration site. Parents at the Demonstration site (where financial charges were waived) reported more satisfaction with the explanation of financial charges than parents at the Comparison site (where parents were required to pay deduction and copayments).

Treatment Planning

Another crucial element of the continuum of care is that treatment is tailored to the individual through coordination by the treatment team. If a child did not have a treatment team meeting, it could be assumed that

Table 4.3. Service Experience with the Intake and Assessment
Process: Percentage Who Reported Receiving Specific Services

Type of service	Demonstration	Comparison
Interview		
Child	94%	80%
Parent	97%	91%
Child		
Physical examination	12%	26%
Psychological tests	15%	36%
Achievement/IQ test	8%	29%
Parent told child's diagnosis	32%	41%
Treatment plan developed	55%	50%
Parent very involved in treatment planning	48%	39%
Financial charges explained	81%	58%

services would be more random and disjointed. Thus, it was important to
determine whether children received services without having had a treatment team meeting. Data indicated that 95% of children who obtained
services at the Demonstration site had a treatment team meeting recorded
in the Management Information System (MIS).[3] It was therefore concluded
that the reason for any failure to produce individualized treatment could
not be that treatment team meetings never occurred. No information about
treatment planning was available through CHAMPUS claims for the Comparison site.

Accuracy of Diagnosis

Using data for children in the Evaluation Sample, clinicians' diagnoses were compared to those determined by the Project's semistructured
diagnostic interviews. Limitations of the diagnoses determined by the
semistructured interviews are discussed in Chapter 2. However, these
interviews provided a way to objectively compare "system-assigned" diagnoses for the sites. Diagnostic categories endorsed for the Evaluation
Sample from the Child Assessment Schedule for Parents (P-CAS) or the
CAS interviews were used as the criteria for comparisons. For the "system-
assigned" (clinicians') diagnoses, all diagnoses provided in the Demonstration MIS or the CHAMPUS data base within a 9-month window

[3]This number differs from the 88.4% reported in the "Use of Intake and Assessment" section
above because this analysis was for individuals who received follow-up services, while the
88.4% represents children who received at least one service, including intake and assessment.

around the date of the Project intake interview (from 6 months prior to 3 months after the collection of Wave 1 data) were used. The 3-month post–Wave 1 period was included to account for the lag time in recording transactions into the two data systems. When "system-assigned" diagnoses were matched to diagnoses determined by the CAS and P-CAS, the two sites performed equally; the percentage of matching diagnoses was less than expected by chance for depression, but greater than expected by chance for the remaining diagnostic categories.

Summary of Utilization Findings

Nine critical utilization issues related to access and to the intake and assessment process were explored in depth in this section. The analyses of seven of these issues indicated strong fidelity to the program model at the Demonstration site and better performance at the Demonstration site than at the Comparison site.

- Access to mental health services increased dramatically at the Demonstration site compared to both the Comparison site and the pre-Demonstration Fort Bragg catchment area time period.
- Community awareness of availability of services and the means by which to access them improved significantly with the implementation of the Demonstration.
- In contrast to the Comparison site, almost all (> 95%) of clients at the Demonstration site received a formal intake and assessment, and there was a low rate of repeated intake–assessments.
- The number and proportion of "one-visit-only" clients was 3 times higher at the Comparison site, highlighting the Demonstration's ability to engage children and families in treatment.
- Timeliness of service delivery following intake and assessment was much better at the Demonstration site.
- Fewer formal evaluation services were used at the Demonstration site, indicating high quality and comprehensiveness of the standardized intake and assessment process.
- Almost all (95%) of clients at the Demonstration site received individualized treatment planning through the treatment team.

In the other two (of nine) areas of utilization examined, findings did not completely support the Demonstration model. The Demonstration and Comparison sites demonstrated equivalent accuracy of diagnosis. In addition, the single point of entry was not completely implemented as planned at the Demonstration site, where some children continued to receive CHAMPUS services. This happened because the Army and the CHAMPUS fiscal intermediary had no formal agreement to disallow CHAMPUS payment for services, even though the services could have been received at the Demonstration site at no charge to parents.

SATISFACTION WITH THE INTAKE
AND ASSESSMENT PROCESS

Consumer views of and satisfaction with intake and assessment procedures were also examined. Parents of children who had been admitted to mental health services at the Demonstration site or the Comparison site were asked to rate various dimensions of the intake and assessment process as part of the Project. Within approximately 30 days of admission to services, parents and children completed a questionnaire about their experiences during the intake and assessment process. The questionnaire measured several dimensions of intake and assessment in addition to providing a global measure of parent satisfaction.

Global Satisfaction

As in most evaluations of consumer satisfaction with services (Stipak, 1980), parents at both the Demonstration site and the Comparison site were generally satisfied with the intake and assessment services they received. Table 4.4 shows that on a scale from 0 (very dissatisfied) to 4 (very satisfied), parents on average responded at or above 3 (satisfied). However, consistently more parents at the Demonstration site (94–98%) than those at the Comparison site (79–86%) reported being satisfied or very satisfied. These differences represent effect sizes favoring the Demonstration site ranging from 0.25 to 0.72 SD.

Dimensions of Satisfaction

As can be seen in Table 4.5, statistically significant differences between the sites were found for ratings of global satisfaction and for 11 of 16 subscales measuring specific dimensions of satisfaction. Parents were significantly more satisfied with intake and assessment services at the Demonstration site in the following areas: access and convenience of location, hours, and the scheduling process; explanation and process of the child and parent interviews during intake; the overall assessment process; involvement in the treatment planning process; the overall process of developing the child's initial treatment plan; relationship with staff, including availability and responsiveness; financial issues, including understanding

Table 4.4. Global Ratings of Parent Satisfaction with the Intake and Assessment Process at Wave 1

Global satisfaction scale item[a]	Demonstration site			Comparison site				
	Mean (SD)	Satisfied[b]	N	Mean (SD)	Satisfied[b]	N	ES	$p(t)$[c]
Did you receive the kind of service you wanted?	3.36[d] (0.63)	94%	506	3.01 (0.78)	79%	386	0.25	<0.01
If a friend were in need of similar help, would you recommend these services?	3.66[d] (0.53)	98%	508	3.19 (0.81)	86%	388	0.72	<0.01
Overall, how satisfied were you with the services you received to date?	3.42[d] (0.62)	94%	509	3.06 (0.77)	85%	384	0.68	<0.01
If you were to seek help again, would you come back to these services?	3.60[d] (0.57)	97%	509	3.15 (0.81)	85%	383	0.67	<0.01
In general, how satisfied were you with the overall intake and assessment process?	3.39[d] (0.62)	95%	500	2.98 (0.75)	82%	386	0.60	<0.01

[a]Global satisfaction questions were adapted from the CSQ-8 (Larsen, Attkisson, Hargreaves, & Nguyen, 1979). Scale: 0 ("very dissatisfied") to 4 ("very satisfied").
[b]Percentage of respondents who endorsed the "satisfied" or "very satisfied" response option.
[c]For t-test of means, Demonstration vs. Comparison.
[d]Statistically significant greater levels of satisfaction at the Demonstration site at $p < 0.01$.

Table 4.5. Parent Satisfaction with the Intake
and Assessment Process at Wave 1

Component of satisfaction	Demonstration site			Comparison site		
	Mean[a]	SD	N[b]	Mean[a]	SD	N[b]
Access and convenience	0.16[c]	0.69	509	−0.20	0.83	396
Child interview	0.14[c]	0.71	466	−0.19	0.93	305
Parent interview	0.17[c]	0.99	487	−0.23	0.98	351
Physical examination	0.10	0.85	60	−0.05	0.94	94
Psychological tests	0.04	0.91	69	−0.03	0.96	132
Achievement/IQ tests	−0.08	1.04	34	0.02	0.91	104
Explanation of diagnosis	0.08	0.95	145	−0.08	1.05	156
Assessment process overall	0.18[c]	0.86	485	−0.24	1.12	358
Involvement in treatment plan	0.12[c]	0.94	275	−0.18	1.05	188
Explanation of treatment plan	0.06	0.90	257	−0.10	1.00	172
Treatment plan process overall	0.12[c]	0.92	276	−0.17	1.09	193
Relationship with staff	0.19[c]	0.73	453	−0.19	0.91	342
Understanding of financial charges	0.18[c]	0.86	402	−0.33	1.15	221
Payment schedule	0.32[c]	0.98	61	−0.19	0.97	104
Amount of payment	0.37[c]	0.68	416	−0.48	1.14	319
Wait for treatment	0.19[c]	0.90	380	−0.24	1.07	291
Global satisfaction	0.25[c]	0.71	495	−0.30	1.00	369

[a]Standardized item scores, which make up each subscale, have a mean of 0. More positive scores
indicate greater satisfaction.
[b]N is the number of parents for whom a subscale could be computed. Some subscales were not
scored if the parent indicated that the corresponding service had not been received.
[c]Statistically significant greater level of satisfaction at the Demonstration site at $p < 0.01$. It was
determined a priori to use the more conservative p-value of <0.01 to indicate significance. For
t-test between means, Demonstration vs. Comparison.

financial charges, the payment schedule, and the amount of payment; and
the wait between the initial request for service and the subsequent availability of treatment services. On the remaining subscales, no significant
differences between sites were found. None of the subscales showed
higher satisfaction ratings at the Comparison site.

Parent Satisfaction with Intake at Different Levels of Care

Parent ratings of satisfaction with intake and assessment at different
levels of care were also assessed. These ratings were categorized according
to the level of restrictiveness of the treatment into which the child was
initially placed. The treatment levels were defined as inpatient hospitalization or RTC, intermediate services (any level of care more than traditional
outpatient and not inpatient or RTC), and traditional outpatient services.
While all three levels of service were available through the Demonstration

site, only the inpatient/RTC and outpatient levels of care were available at the Comparison site. Thus, only results of analyses on these two levels of care are examined below.

Parent ratings were analyzed from two perspectives. First, within-site comparisons were conducted individually for each site (to assess the degree to which different levels of care were associated with differences in parents' ratings of satisfaction). Second, between-site comparisons were conducted within the same treatment level (to assess the extent to which parents' ratings of satisfaction of the same level of care differed between the Demonstration and Comparison sites).

Within-Site, Across Levels of Care

As noted earlier, all three levels of care were available at the Demonstration site. However, due to limited sample sizes in the intermediate levels of care, within-site comparisons were restricted to inpatient/RTC and outpatient services. Means for the different levels of care for the Demonstration and Comparison sites are presented in Table 4.6. One component of the intake and assessment process at the Demonstration site was rated differently depending on level of service (as indicated by footnote d, corresponding to the level of care with the highest rating). Significantly greater satisfaction was expressed with achievement and IQ testing at intake into outpatient services than at intake into inpatient/RTC services. Other mean differences for components of the intake and assessment process were not statistically significant.

For the Comparison site, only the most and least restrictive levels of care were available, and there were few differences in parent ratings of satisfaction based on level of care. Parents whose children were placed in inpatient or residential facilities tended to be more satisfied with three aspects of the intake and assessment process than parents of children receiving outpatient services. Parents of children placed in the most restrictive levels of care reported significantly more satisfaction with access and convenience, their relationships with staff, and the assessment process overall than did parents of children in outpatient settings.

Between-Site, Within Similar Levels of Care

In the second stage of analysis, also reported in Table 4.6, comparisons were made between sites within the same level of treatment restrictiveness. These comparisons were conducted only for the most and least restrictive levels of care (inpatient/RTC and outpatient), as the intermediate levels of care were available only at the Demonstration site.

Table 4.6. Parent Satisfaction with the Intake and Assessment Process at Wave 1 across Different Levels of Care[a]

Component of satisfaction	Demonstration site[b]		Comparison site[b]	
	Inpatient mean (SD) (N = 54)	Outpatient mean (SD) (N = 391)	Inpatient mean (SD) (N = 31)	Outpatient mean (SD) (N = 177)
Access and convenience	0.31 (0.71)[c]	0.16 (0.66)[c]	−0.02 (0.78)[d]	−0.26 (0.83)
Child interview	0.14 (0.66)	0.14 (0.72)[c]	−0.09 (0.90)	−0.24 (0.94)
Parent interview	0.15 (0.93)	0.23 (0.93)[c]	−0.12 (0.97)	−0.27 (0.98)
Physical examination	0.24 (0.80)	0.03 (0.89)	−0.12 (1.08)	0.03 (0.75)
Psychological tests	−0.06 (0.86)	0.21 (0.91)	0.15 (1.09)	0.08 (0.83)
Achievement/IQ tests	−0.42 (0.97)	0.79 (0.34)[c,d]	−0.13 (1.04)	0.14 (0.78)
Explanation of diagnosis	0.00 (0.93)	0.14 (0.98)	−0.10 (1.18)	−0.06 (0.96)
Assessment process overall	0.03 (0.78)	0.22 (0.85)[c]	0.00 (1.07)[d]	−0.33 (1.12)
Involvement in treatment plan	0.10 (0.94)	0.16 (0.93)[c]	−0.21 (1.16)	−0.16 (0.98)
Explanation of treatment plan	0.07 (0.83)	0.09 (0.90)	−0.11 (1.09)	−0.09 (0.95)
Treatment plan process overall	0.12 (0.90)	0.13 (0.90)[c]	−0.11 (1.08)	−0.21 (1.10)
Relationship with staff	0.20 (0.75)	0.23 (0.69)[c]	0.00 (0.92)[d]	−0.27 (0.89)
Understanding of financial charges	−0.09 (1.12)	0.23 (0.81)[c]	−0.33 (1.19)	−0.33 (1.12)
Payment schedule	−0.18 (1.52)	0.40 (0.90)[c]	−0.20 (0.89)	−0.18 (1.02)
Amount of payment	0.33 (0.59)[c]	0.38 (0.68)[c]	−0.62 (1.09)	−0.41 (1.16)
Wait for treatment	0.31 (0.81)	0.23 (0.89)[c]	−0.04 (1.03)	−0.34 (1.08)
Global satisfaction	0.28 (0.68)[c]	0.29 (0.66)[c]	−0.19 (1.01)	−0.35 (1.00)

[a]Parents' ratings of the intake and assessment process were compared across the service settings in which their children received the intake and assessment services.

[b]Means were based on the number of respondents whose children utilized each service component, resulting in different Ns for each mean. Ns at the Demonstration site ranged from 8 for Payment schedule to 54 for Parent interview in the Inpatient category and from 8 for Achievement/IQ tests to 391 for Access and convenience in the Outpatient category. Ns at the Comparison sites ranged from 11 for Understanding financial charges to 31 for Global satisfaction in the Inpatient category and from 26 for Achievement/IQ tests to 177 for Access and convenience in the Outpatient category. Items within each subscale reported were standardized to a mean of 0 across a polled sample of both sites and all levels of care. More positive ratings indicate greater satisfaction.

[c]Between-site comparisons revealed significant differences in a t-test of means between Demonstration and Comparison, within a single level of care, at $p < 0.01$.

[d]Within-site comparisons revealed significant differences, across different levels of care, at $p < 0.01$, based on a t-test between two levels of care.

In the context of an inpatient residential setting, parents at the Demonstration site reported greater satisfaction than Comparison site parents in the following areas: access and convenience, the amount of financial charges for which they were responsible, and overall global satisfaction with the intake and assessment process. It is notable that parents at the

Demonstration site reported greater satisfaction globally and with those areas of the inpatient intake and assessment process most directly influenced by the Demonstration site: access and convenience and amount of payment. It should be noted that inpatient services were delivered through contracted inpatient hospitals. In the other 14 areas, where inpatient facilities operated more independently of such influence, reports of satisfaction were similar between sites.

Parent ratings of satisfaction with intake and assessment in the context of outpatient services for their children revealed that differences between the Demonstration and Comparison sites cut across most aspects of the intake and assessment process. In all but four areas, parents at the Demonstration site reported significantly greater satisfaction with services than parents at the Comparison site.

Summary of Parent Satisfaction with Intake to Different Levels of Care

Parent ratings of satisfaction with the intake and assessment process were examined to determine the degree to which differences in levels of satisfaction were associated with children's assignment to different levels of care (inpatient/RTC or outpatient services). Analyses were conducted both within-site, across different levels of care, and between sites, within the same level of care. The Demonstration site received higher ratings of parent satisfaction in most aspects of the intake and assessment process.

ACCESS AND THE INTAKE AND ASSESSMENT PROCESS: SUMMARY

The intake and assessment process is an integral part of the continuum-of-care concept. One important feature of the Demonstration model was a single point of entry into the continuum of care, allowing for a central, standardized, and coordinated intake process. The Demonstration implemented such a single point of entry with both fidelity to its proposed model and high quality. In contrast, at the Comparison site, neither a single point of entry nor a standardized intake and assessment procedure was uniformly in place. The effects of these differing methods for accessing child and adolescent mental health care were analyzed on the basis of ratings by community experts, utilization patterns, and reports of satisfaction with services.

When community experts were asked to rate mental health services for military dependents in their communities, they reported significantly greater adequacy and quality of the intake and assessment process at the Demonstration site. On items assessing service system performance regarding access to mental health care, the Demonstration site also received significantly more positive ratings.

Nine critical utilization issues related to access and the intake and assessment process were explored in depth in this section. The analyses of seven of these issues indicated strong fidelity to the program model at the Demonstration site and better performance at the Demonstration site than at the Comparison site. In the other two areas of utilization examined, findings did not fully support the model of the Demonstration.

The Demonstration site received significantly higher ratings of parent satisfaction than the Comparison site on global ratings of the intake and assessment process and on 11 of 16 subscales measuring specific dimensions of satisfaction. These findings support the program theory that ease of access, reduced financial burden, and the individualized assessment process at the Demonstration site should lead to increased consumer satisfaction.

5

The Treatment Process and Service Utilization

Mental health treatment involves the critical process of providing the appropriate service to children once they have accessed care and have participated in initial assessment as described in Chapter 4. To meet children's mental health needs most appropriately, the Demonstration proposed to provide a wide variety of services within a comprehensive and coordinated continuum of care, providing the best opportunity for matching children's needs to services. Figure 1.1 is reproduced as Figure 5.1 to present the components of the program theory model related to treatment.

This chapter describes the treatment processes at the Demonstration and Comparison sites. Ratings of the adequacy, quality, and service system performance are presented. Next, service utilization and patterns of treatment are addressed. Consumer views of their satisfaction with treatment processes at the Demonstration and Comparison sites are presented. Finally, a discussion of the quality of the system of care, in terms of appropriateness of treatment, is presented.

DESCRIPTION OF TREATMENT

Treatment at the Demonstration Site

The Demonstration provided a clear an unambiguous structure and treatment philosophy. Structurally, the services at the Demonstration site were delivered through a continuum of care that provided a comprehensive range of services. At the extreme ends of the continuum, reflecting the least and most restrictive levels of care, respectively, were outpatient ser-

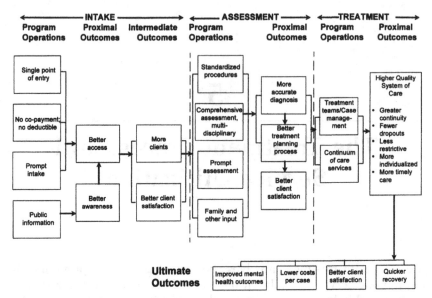

Figure 5.1. Fort Bragg Child and Adolescent Demonstration: Program theory.

vices and inpatient psychiatric hospitalization. Both these levels of care were provided through contracts with existing community providers and organizations. In addition, contract services were available through a residential treatment center (RTC). These types of services had been traditionally reimbursed through the Civilian Health and Medical Program of the Uniformed Services (CHAMPUS) and were available in the community prior to the Demonstration, as they were at the Comparison site.

The intermediate levels of service, however, were a unique contribution of the Demonstration. Services offered 24 hours a day included therapeutic group homes and therapeutic homes. Several levels of intensive day services were also provided. Also available around the clock was in-home crisis stabilization, through which clients could access a range of services designed to maintain a child within the family home when there was a high risk of out-of-home placement. Day treatment and partial hospitalization provided specialized mental health care and educational treatment 5 days per week. Within the Rumbaugh Clinic, intensive outpatient and evaluation services were provided. In addition, wraparound services were available to clients in any of the levels of care, if specified in the treatment plan.

In addition to many levels of care, the Demonstration developed a mechanism for assessing client needs for placement in the most appropriate setting and for moving the client in a timely and planned manner when a change to a more or less restrictive treatment was indicated.

Initial assessment during the intake process was described in Chapter 4. In summary, the Rumbaugh Clinic served as the single point of entry for the target population. Referrals were screened for eligibility and emergency status, and a comprehensive standardized intake and assessment process was conducted for routine admission. Once a child was in treatment, the case management and treatment teams provided this mechanism.

The treatment philosophy of the Demonstration clearly stated its plan to be an individualized, community-based, family-focused system of care (as represented in the program theory model in Figure 5.1). In essence:

> The continuum of care approach is child-centered and family-focused. Services are designed and "wrapped around" the child and family, instead of expecting the family to conform to the existing system. Care is delivered in the least restrictive setting possible (Cardinal Mental Health Group, 1990a).

These philosophical goals are considered the desired, but nevertheless hard to achieve, state of the art in children's mental health services, as promoted by the Child and Adolescent Service System Program. There is much documentation regarding the description and implementation of the structural facets of the Demonstration, so these aspects will not be reviewed here in detail.[1] As noted above, the intake and assessment process was described in Chapter 4. The specific treatment components (outpatient, day treatment, in-home crisis stabilization, group home and other residential, and acute inpatient) as well as the coordinating mechanisms of case management and treatment teams are described in depth in program documents. However, one aspect of the program, the Utilization Review and Management (UR/M) process, will be highlighted here because of its impact on service utilization at the Demonstration site and, consequently, on system costs.

Utilization Review and Management at the Demonstration Site

The Demonstration was a test of the theory that clinical judgments of appropriateness and quality of services would contain costs better than "arbitrary" limits on services or expenditures (Behar et al., 1995). Soon

---

[1]See Behar (1992) for a description of fully implemented services. See the Interim Report of the Fort Bragg Evaluation Project (1991) and the final report of the Implementation Study of the Fort Bragg Evaluation Project (Heflinger, 1993) for detailed information on the activities involved in all phases of implementing the services of the Demonstration.

after the Demonstration began, the Rumbaugh Clinic and the Army began discussion of issues related to service utilization and costs.

Although the Rumbaugh Clinic was not required to meet the standards of the Joint Commission on Accreditation of Health Care Organizations for utilization review (UR), it did record and report service utilization and workload data on a fairly regular basis (Heflinger, 1993). A Utilization Management Team was created and, by June 1992, a Utilization Management Plan was developed. As the plan became effective, Cardinal, the State, and the Army expressed concerns about service utilization and costs during Project Oversight Committee meetings; Cardinal and the State recommended more rigorous review of more-than-outpatient services, while the Health Services Command eliminated the Rumbaugh Clinic's Outpatient Care Coordinators.

In January 1994, the Army completed a review of the Rumbaugh Clinic's Quality Improvement (QI)/Risk Management (RM)/Utilization Management (UM) Plan and its implementation (Hostetter, 1994). While the QI and RM components satisfied reviewers, the UM Plan was faulted for several deficiencies:

- It substituted data collection for data analysis.
- Collected data were not adequately transformed into cost data and thus were not incorporated into treatment decisions as the UM plan and program theory required.
- The UM process was not adequately coordinated.

An independent evaluator[2] and a State reviewer[3] also noted problems with the Rumbaugh Clinic's monitoring, evaluation, and analytical activities. Clearly, the Demonstration developed a system for monitoring and utilizing information about service utilization and costs. However, the system apparently was not refined and made fully operational quickly enough to achieve its goal of replacing arbitrary CHAMPUS limits on services with more clinically meaningful limits based on empirical findings.[4]

[2]See Bickman et al. (1993) for a review conducted by Sequest Health Care Systems, Inc.
[3]Michael Schwartz of MH/DD/SAS prepared a memo to Dr. Lenore Behar stating his impressions of Cardinal's UR/M process and assessing the possibility of the State's preparing Cardinal's monthly reports.
[4]Project Oversight Committee meeting minutes and utilization review documents and reports; correspondence between North Carolina, Cardinal, and the Army; and previous reviews by Vanderbilt Project staff comprised the bulk of documentation for this limited review. Documentation produced by Rumbaugh's Clinical Management Teams and information about the Rumbaugh Clinic's use of the Pioneer Unit Cost Findings were not included, as they were not available to Project staff.

Treatment at the Comparison Site

In contrast to the Demonstration site, only the traditional and extreme ends of the continuum of care (outpatient services, RTCs, and inpatient hospitalization) were available to CHAMPUS-eligible children at the Comparison site. As previously discussed, mental health benefits available under CHAMPUS changed in October 1990. Precertification of RTC and inpatient hospital admissions limited treatment.

Children and families at the Comparison site could access treatment in one of three ways. They could use their CHAMPUS benefits for outpatient, RTC, or inpatient treatment, subject to the limits mentioned above. They could seek outpatient services available through the on-post hospital. Last, they could go outside the CHAMPUS system by using other insurance benefits. Families who chose to use the last option were outside the CHAMPUS–Army network and the Project. Information was available to the Project, however, to describe the first two options.

A loosely coupled network of CHAMPUS providers existed in the communities surrounding both Comparison-site posts. At Fort Campbell, outpatient service providers were located in Clarksville, Tennessee, and Hopkinsville, Kentucky, each approximately 15 minutes from the post, and in Nashville, Tennessee, 1 hour away. Treatment in RTCs and inpatient facilities was available in those communities as well as in Dickson, Tennessee, 30 minutes away. Near Fort Stewart, a smaller choice of outpatient providers was available in Hinesville, Georgia; within a 45-minute drive, a broader range of outpatient and inpatient providers was available in Savannah and Brunswick, Georgia. The closest RTC to Fort Stewart was several hours away, however, and appeared to be used more as a step-down service for inpatient hospitalization than as an initial or unique treatment option (as RTC treatment was used at Fort Campbell).

As described in Chapter 4, access to mental health services became more limited at the Comparison site during the course of the Project as Gateway to Care was implemented. Fort Campbell personnel screened admissions to outpatient services and RTCs, at least informally, in addition to having a formal requirement of obtaining a Nonavailability of Service (NAS) form from the psychiatry clinic for inpatient hospitalization. This NAS procedure was also instituted at Fort Stewart. In addition, a precertification process provided by Health Management Strategies International, Inc. (HMS) was required at both sites.

Both Comparison-site locations offered, at some level, outpatient services to children and families on post and at no cost. During calendar years 1992 (at Fort Campbell) and 1993 (at Fort Stewart), Army personnel were more available for this option than at other times.

However, no other intermediate-level services were available through CHAMPUS or on post; children in outpatient services in need of more intensive treatment were faced with the options of an RTC or inpatient hospitalization. Likewise, children in these more restrictive levels of care had access only to psychotherapy in the community when they were discharged. Coordination between providers and levels of care was dependent on the level of interest and resources of the involved providers, since no formal coordinating mechanism existed.

A limited model of case management was implemented at Fort Campbell in mid-1992. A case manager was hired to network with the area RTCs and hospitals and encouraged shorter lengths of stay and use of other local resources. However, unlike case managers at the Demonstration site, this case manager had no authority or formal relationship with the treatment facilities. Although he maintained contact with these facilities, the HMS process for pre-certifying and authorizing payment for specified numbers of days was the main determinant of length of stay.

In summary, the Demonstration site provided a variety of treatment types and intensities and a mechanism for monitoring and adapting service delivery. At the Comparison site, services were limited to traditional outpatient care and residential treatment (inpatient hospitals and RTCs). Services at the Comparison site were not linked by formal case management, as they were at the Demonstration site. The effects of these differing models of service delivery were examined through ratings by community experts, utilization patterns, and reports of satisfaction with services.

RATINGS BY COMMUNITY EXPERTS

As part of the Implementation Study (Heflinger, 1993), community experts responded to a written survey assessing adequacy, quality, and service system performance of the mental health system for military dependents. These community experts included psychologists, psychiatrists, social workers, school and juvenile court personnel, and Army personnel. As can be seen in Table 5.1, experts rated the *adequacy* of mental health services at the Demonstration site as significantly greater than that at the Comparison site for all eight service types. Similarly, as can be seen in Table 5.2, the *quality* of all eight types of mental health services was rated significantly higher at the Demonstration site. Table 5.3 shows that among the service *system performance* items rated significantly better at the Demonstration site, those receiving the highest ratings at the Demonstration site were providing services at reasonable costs to families, using written treatment plans, encouraging treatment options to children in community-

Table 5.1. Community Ratings of Mental Health Services
for Military Dependent Children: Adequacy

Type of mental health service	Demonstration site			Comparison site				
	Mean[a]	SD	N	Mean[a]	SD	N	ES	$p(t)$[b]
Outpatient mental health services	4.25[c]	0.61	44	3.35	0.90	67	1.15	<0.01
Emergency services	4.12[c]	0.79	43	3.40	1.02	62	0.78	<0.01
Case management	4.02[c]	1.02	46	3.01	0.96	59	1.02	<0.01
Inpatient/residential treatment	3.88[c]	0.82	43	3.20	0.98	69	0.74	<0.01
Substance abuse services	3.67[c]	0.81	39	3.10	0.92	59	0.65	<0.01
Day treatment/partial hospitalization	3.66[c]	0.88	41	2.34	1.00	58	1.33	<0.01
Other residential mental health services	3.56[c]	0.85	43	2.47	0.77	59	1.36	<0.01
In-home services	3.55[c]	0.83	42	2.21	0.87	52	1.58	<0.01

[a]Scale: 1 ("very poor") to 5 ("very good").
[b]From a *t*-test between means, Demonstration vs. Comparison site.
[c]Significantly better performance at the Demonstration site than at the Comparison site at $p < 0.01$.

Table 5.2. Community Ratings of Mental Health Services
for Military Dependent Children: Quality

Type of mental health service	Demonstration site			Comparison site				
	Mean[a]	SD	N	Mean[a]	SD	N	ES	$p(t)$[b]
Outpatient mental health services	4.24[c]	0.61	45	3.32	1.13	65	1.00	<0.01
Emergency services	4.21[c]	0.74	43	3.19	1.23	57	1.00	<0.01
Case management	4.02[c]	1.06	43	2.94	0.94	47	1.09	<0.01
Inpatient/residential treatment	3.64[c]	0.89	44	3.00	1.14	64	0.62	<0.01
Substance abuse services	3.93[c]	0.83	43	3.23	1.02	57	0.74	<0.01
Day treatment/partial hospitalization	3.95[c]	0.85	40	2.51	1.06	45	1.5	<0.01
Other residential mental health services	3.77[c]	0.90	43	2.42	0.89	53	1.5	<0.01
In-home services	4.00[c]	0.87	43	2.32	1.04	41	1.8	<0.01

[a]Scale: 1 ("very poor") to 5 ("very good").
[b]From a *t*-test between means, Demonstration vs. Comparison site.
[c]Significantly better performance at the Demonstration site than at the Comparison site at $p < 0.01$.

Table 5.3. Community Ratings of Mental Health Services for Military Dependent Children: System Performance

Service system performance	Mean[a]	
	Demonstration ($N = 47$)	Comparison ($N = 67$)
Providing services at reasonable cost to families	4.62[b]	3.02
Using written treatment plans that include goals, planned services, frequency of service, specific objectives, and dates to accomplish them	4.61[b]	3.21
Encouraging options for treatment of children in community-based settings	4.33[b]	2.64
Making appropriate mental health services available to all children and their families who need them	4.27[b]	2.75
Offering high-quality mental health treatment services	4.20[b]	3.03
Tailoring services to special needs of children and their families	4.20[b]	2.62
Providing children and their families with services that consider their individual needs and strengths	4.13[b]	2.76
Integrating diagnostic and treatment services for children with both mental health and substance abuse problems	4.10[b]	2.87
Expanding service capability to meet growing needs of children and their families 2.59		4.09[b]
Encouraging parents to become actively involved in the treatment of their children	4.04[b]	3.08
Ensuring that children are placed in the most appropriate service setting	4.04[b]	2.81
Making supportive services available to all children and their families who need them	3.95[b]	2.68
Coordinating services across agencies to meet the individual needs of children and their families	3.86[b]	2.45
Ensuring meaningful discharge planning between inpatient psychiatric centers and community-based mental health services	3.70[b]	2.56
Ensuring that all agencies and providers have timely access to client records in ways that do not violate client confidentiality/rights	3.64[b]	2.65
Establishing adequate grievance mechanisms for children and their families	3.62[b]	2.17
Providing transportation to services/events when needed	3.46[b]	1.95
Ensuring that children who reach age 18 are transmitted into adult services smoothly	3.31[b]	2.39
Ensuring that children who lose their eligibility for CHAMPUS continue to receive services	2.57[b]	2.16

[a]Scale: 1 ("very poor") to 5 ("very good"). Means for each component were based on the total number of respondents for each item, which ranged from 26 to 47 at the Demonstration site and from 33 to 67 at the Comparison site.
[b]Significantly better mental health service system performance at the Demonstration site than at the Comparison site (using t-test between means) at $p < 0.01$.

based settings, and making appropriate mental health services available to all children and their families who needed them.

SERVICE UTILIZATION

Literature on mental health services utilization suggests that efforts to measure differences focus on five dimensions of service use: type, mix, volume, distribution over time, and continuity of services received. Thus, utilization of services during the treatment phase should have differed in tangible ways between sites. Each of the five treatment dimensions is discussed below; differences between the Demonstration and Comparison sites during the Demonstration period[5] are presented. Actual differences between sites (not estimates) are reported. Unless noted, all tables and figures present data for the treated population; since these figures, then, represent a census, measures of statistical significance are inappropriate.[6]

Type of Service Received

This dimension recognizes that mental health services are provided in a variety of settings. Thus, it is important to characterize not only whether a child was treated but also the *type* of service he or she received (Dorken, 1977; Leaf & Bruce, 1987). Clearly, more children received services at the Demonstration site, as described in the section regarding access in Chapter 4, but three questions remain: What services did they receive? Were the new services made available by the Demonstration used by a significant proportion of clients? Were more clients using the services than had traditionally used them under CHAMPUS? Table 5.4 characterizes the types of services received by presenting the proportion of treated children who received services in each of several settings.

Traditional care under CHAMPUS was a mix of inpatient hospitalization, RTCs, and outpatient therapy. Table 5.4 shows that prior to the Demonstration, the types of services provided at the sites were quite similar. Roughly 1 in 6 children (15–18%) treated in a given fiscal year were hospitalized; fewer than 1 in 20 (1–6%) were treated in RTCs. More than 4 of 5 (>80%) received outpatient therapy. Prior to the Demonstration period, the only way that sites differed was that children treated at the Comparison site were more likely to be placed in an RTC.

The Demonstration had a conspicuous effect on the treatment children received. Intermediate-level services (e.g., therapeutic group homes)

---

[5]The Demonstration period for the Utilization and Cost Studies is defined as October 1, 1990, through September 30, 1993.
[6]See Harnett (1980) for a discussion of the difference between a sample and a population.

Table 5.4. Mix of Services: Number of Children Receiving Service of a Given Type and Those Children as a Percentage of All Treated Children

Period	Hospital	RTC	Intermediate residential	Intermediate nonresidential	Outpatient	Assessment and evaluation	Case management	Treatment team
	Number of children and percentage of treated children receiving each service[a]							
Demonstration site								
Fiscal year								
1988 (N = 938)	152 16.2%	19 2.0%	NA	NA	808 86.1%	496 52.9%	NA	NA
1989 (N = 1124)	176 15.7%	18 1.6%	NA	NA	923 82.1%	522 46.4%	NA	NA
1990				Transition period				
1991 (N = 2648)	197 7.4%	45 1.7%	87 3.3%	134 5.1%	2246 84.8%	2018 76.2%	629 23.8%	1541 58.2%
1992 (N = 3327)	238 7.2%	25 0.8%	176 5.3%	289 8.7%	2856 85.8%	2068 62.2%	760 22.8%	2217 66.6%
1993 (N = 3572)	181 5.1%	6 0.2%	200 5.6%	241 6.7%	3079 86.2%	2280 63.8%	452 12.7%	2370 66.3%
Demonstration period[b] (N = 6033)	501 8.3%	70 1.2%	341 5.7%	495 8.2%	5249 87.0%	5507 91.3%	1342 22.2%	5136 85.1%
Comparison site								
Fiscal year								
1988 (N = 949)	172 18.1%	57 6.0%	NA	NA	794 83.7%	460 48.5%	NA	NA
1989 (N = 1189)	185 15.6%	55 4.6%	NA	NA	969 81.5%	598 50.3%	NA	NA
1990 (N = 1242)	212 17.1%	61 4.9%	NA	NA	1008 81.2%	508 40.9%	NA	NA
1991 (N= 1322)	236 17.9%	50 3.8%	NA	NA	1126 85.2%	623 47.1%	NA	NA
1992 (N = 1108)	103 9.3%	30 2.7%	NA	NA	955 86.2%	481 43.4%	NA	NA
1993 (N = 1145)	99 8.6%	29 2.5%	NA	NA	1002 87.5%	598 52.2%	NA	NA
Demonstration period[b] (N = 2780)	396 14.2%	91 3.3%	NA	NA	2414 86.8%	1537 55.3%	NA	NA

[a]These data describe the treated population at the Comparison and Demonstration sites. Each entry indicates the number and percentage of children treated during a given period who received the particular type of service. For example, 16.2% of children treated in the Demonstration site catchment area were hospitalized in fiscal year 1988.

[b]The Demonstration period is the combined fiscal years 1991–1993.

were unavailable under CHAMPUS, but were provided to fairly large numbers of children under the Demonstration. A total of 341 children received intermediate residential services at the Demonstration site during the Demonstration period. This number represents over 5% of children treated and is nearly as many as were hospitalized. Nearly 1 in 12 children treated received care in an intermediate nonresidential setting. In addition, considerable effort was expended to make sure that the right children received the new intermediate-level services and that these services were integrated with others. Over one fifth of children treated during the Demonstration period had case management. Similarly, treatment teams met to discuss more than 85% of all cases and 95% of the cases of children who received services after the intake and assessment process.

Clearly, the Demonstration made new services available. According to proponents of the continuum-of-care model, providing intermediate-level services should reduce use of other more restrictive services. The proportion of children treated in a hospital or RTC was considerably lower at the Demonstration site. Only 8% of children treated at the Demonstration site were hospitalized, and just over 1% were placed in RTCs. These percentages are much lower than for the Fort Bragg catchment area prior to the Demonstration or for the Comparison site. The likelihood that a treated child would be hospitalized at the Comparison site (14%) was 75% higher than at the Demonstration site.

From fiscal year 1991 to fiscal year 1993, the use of hospitalization and RTCs fell dramatically at the Comparison site. Nonetheless, the likelihood that a treated child would be hospitalized was still considerably lower at the Demonstration site than at the Comparison site in fiscal year 1993.

Mix of Services Received

Measures of how many children received a given service (e.g., outpatient therapy) do not account for the mix of services a given child received. Two aspects of service mix were especially important in light of the goals of the program theory of the Demonstration: the most restrictive setting in which a child was treated and the services that were combined with intermediate services.

Most Restrictive Service

While the concept of restrictiveness of care is multi-dimensional (Bachrach, 1980; Carpenter, 1978), focus generally centers on the setting of care, with inpatient services or other out-of-home placements representing "more restrictive" services and partial hospitalization and office visits representing "less restrictive" services (Bickman, Heflinger, Pion, & Behar, 1991; Burns, 1991; Ranshoff, Zachary, Gaynor, & Hargreaves, 1982).

Table 5.5 shows the most restrictive service that children received (in order from most to least restrictive): inpatient hospitalization, RTC, intermediate residential, intermediate nonresidential, and outpatient therapy.

Prior to the Demonstration, nearly 4 of 5 children (80%) treated in a given fiscal year received services in the least restrictive setting, outpatient therapy. This proportion was somewhat higher in the Fort Bragg catchment area because children there were much less likely to be admitted to an RTC. The Demonstration "moved" children away from both ends of the spectrum of restrictiveness. Children were less likely to be treated in a hospital or RTC after the Demonstration began, and at the same time, the proportion of children who received only outpatient treatment fell in fiscal year 1991 and fiscal year 1992. These data indicate that the intermediate services drew children from both groups, although those likely to have been placed in a hospital or RTC appear to have contributed more heavily to increased utilization of intermediate services.

The additional services offered under the Demonstration moved individuals toward the middle of the spectrum of restrictiveness, as would be predicted on the basis of the program theory. Under traditional CHAMPUS coverage at the Comparison site, children were concentrated at the two ends of the spectrum, needing either outpatient therapy or hospitalization. Table 5.5 also shows, however, that use of hospitalization fell at the Comparison site during fiscal year 1992 and fiscal year 1993. Without the availability of intermediate services, these children were moved into outpatient services only or even out of services altogether.

Use of Intermediate Services

Another way of characterizing service mix is to examine the way in which the intermediate services were combined with services in more restrictive settings. This dimension seems particularly relevant in light of the program theory of the Demonstration. Since these services should enable children to leave care in more restrictive settings, they should be targeted to children with more severe problems. Table 5.6 demonstrates that case management, treatment team services, and care in intermediate settings are targeted to children with the most severe problems. Children who received case management during the Demonstration period, for example, were over 20 times as likely to have been hospitalized (32.0%) as children who did not receive those services (1.5%). Similarly, children who received treatment team services and care in intermediate settings were much more likely to have been hospitalized.

Table 5.5. Restrictiveness: Percentage of Children Receiving Their Most Restrictive Service by Year[a]

Period	Hospital	RTC	Intermediate residential	Intermediate nonresidential	Outpatient	Other
Demonstration site						
Fiscal year						
1988 (N = 938)	16.2%	1.0%	NA	NA	79.1%	3.7%
1989 (N = 1124)	15.7%	1.1%	NA	NA	79.1%	4.2%
1990				Transition period		
1991 (N = 2648)	7.4%	0.8%	1.3%	17.3%	73.1%	0.1%
1992 (N = 3327)	7.2%	0.2%	2.7%	15.2%	74.8%	<0.1%
1993 (N = 3572)	5.1%	<0.1%	3.4%	5.9%	85.6%	<0.1%
Demonstration period[b] (N = 6033)	8.3%	0.3%	2.4%	14.2%	75.1%	<0.1%
Comparison site						
Fiscal year						
1988 (N = 949)	18.1%	5.2%	NA	NA	74.7%	2.0%
1989 (N = 1189)	15.6%	4.1%	NA	NA	78.3%	2.0%
1990 (N = 1242)	17.1%	3.6%	NA	NA	75.8%	3.5%
1991 (N = 1322)	17.9%	2.6%	NA	NA	76.3%	3.3%
1992 (N = 1108)	9.3%	1.9%	NA	NA	86.3%	2.5%
1993 (N = 1145)	8.6%	1.3%	NA	NA	88.4%	1.7%
Demonstration period[b] (N = 2780)	14.2%	1.5%	NA	NA	82.1%	2.2%

[a]These data describe the treated population at the Comparison and Demonstration sites. Each entry indicates the most restrictive care a child treated in a given period received. Of the children treated at the Demonstration site in fiscal year 1988, for example, 16.2% were treated in a hospital.
[b]The Demonstration period is the combined fiscal years 1991–1993.

Table 5.6. Relationship between Intermediate and Residential Services at the Demonstration Site: Likelihood That a Child Receiving Case Management or Other Intermediate Services Would Be Hospitalized or Placed in a Residential Treatment Center (Demonstration Period Only)[a]

	Received:							
	Case management? (N = 6033)		Treatment team? (N = 6033)		Intermediate residential? (N = 6033)		Intermediate nonresidential? (N = 6033)	
Treatment	Yes (1342)	No (4691)	Yes (5136)	No (897)	Yes (341)	No (5692)	Yes (495)	No (5538)
Admitted to hospital	32.0%	1.5%	8.9%	5.0%	57.2%	5.4%	52.5%	4.0%
Treated in RTC	4.0%	0.4%	1.2%	0.8%	11.1%	5.6%	8.7%	0.5%
Treated in intermediate residential settings	22.4%	0.8%	6.2%	2.6%	—		40.1%	2.5%

[a]These data describe the treated population at the Demonstration site. The Demonstration period is the combined fiscal years 1991–1993. The entries in each pair of columns indicate the treatments received by children who did or did not receive the service specified by the subhead over that pair. The entries in the first column, for example, indicate the treatments received by the 1342 children who received case management. The entries in each row indicate the percentages of children who received the service named in that row. For example, 32.0% of children who received case management were admitted to a hospital at some point during the Demonstration period.

It appears, therefore, that the services added under the Demonstration were targeted to the most severe cases, as indicated by the increased likelihood that they were provided to children who also were hospitalized or treated in RTCs. Table 5.7 suggests that in addition, significant proportions of children hospitalized or treated in an RTC received these other services. Of children hospitalized, more than 85% received case management, and 7 of 10 received an intermediate service.

Volume of Services Received

Measures of volume (or "dose") define a unit of treatment for each type of service and simply tabulate those units. One might count, for example, total number of inpatient days or outpatient visits (Dorken, VandenBos, Cummings, & Pallak, 1993; Rice, Kelman, Miller, & Dunmeyer, 1990) or calculate the mean number of services received. Change in average number of visits or hospital days is a popular measure of utilization of mental health services (Patrick et al., 1993; Tsai et al., 1988). The following

Table 5.7. Relationship between Intermediate and Residential Services at the Demonstration Site: Likelihood That a Child Hospitalized or Placed in a Residential Treatment Center Would Receive Case Management or Other Intermediate Service (Demonstration Period Only)[a]

Service	Hospitalized? (N = 6033)		Treated in TCR? (N = 6033)		Treated in intermediate residential facility? (N = 6033)	
	Yes (501)	No (5532)	Yes (70)	No (5963)	Yes (341)	No (5692)
Receiving case management	85.8%	16.5%	75.7%	21.6%	88.0%	18.3%
With treatment team services	91.0%	84.6%	90.0%	85.1%	93.3%	84.7%
With intermediate residential	38.9%	3.7%	54.3%	5.1%	—	—
With intermediate nonresidential	51.9%	4.3%	61.4%	2.6%	59.2%	5.2%

[a]These data describe the treated population at the Demonstration site. The Demonstration period is the combined fiscal years 1991–1993. The entries in each pair of columns indicate the treatments received by children who did or did not receive the service specified by the subhead over that pair. The entries in the first column, for example, indicate the treatments received by the 501 children who were hospitalized. The entries in each row indicate the percentages of children who received the service named in that row. For example, 85.8% of children who received case management were admitted to a hospital at some point during the Demonstration period.

discussion presents the mean number of service encounters for each category of services.[7] Inpatient hospitalization and use of RTCs are a focus, since they involve placement out of the home. Several measures centering on these two most restrictive settings are presented and include average number of days hospitalized children spent out of home, average length of stay (LOS), average number of admissions for each child hospitalized, and total days spent out of home. The discussion uses each of these measures to judge whether, overall, the Demonstration reduced use of out-of-home placements.

Table 5.8 reveals that prior to the Demonstration, there were some differences in service use between the two sites. Children receiving outpatient therapy in fiscal years 1988 or 1989 had roughly 6 visits over the course of the year, and children at the Comparison site had approximately 1 more visit per year, on average, than children at the Demonstration site. Children in the Fort Bragg catchment area who were hospitalized at some point during fiscal years 1988 or 1989 spent, on average, 35 days out of home (roughly 1 week less than children at the Comparison site during the same time period). Children who received care in RTCs before the Demonstration period in the Fort Bragg catchment area spent, on average, over 18 weeks out of home. This number is strikingly higher than that for hospitalization and likely reflects the fact that CHAMPUS has historically limited hospitalization more stringently than care in RTCs. The gap between days out of home for hospitalization and RTC treatment is even larger for the Comparison site, where children treated in RTCs spent over half the year out of home.

Table 5.8 shows that during the Demonstration period, in contrast, the average number of hospital days was about the same between sites, while the average number of days in RTC at the Demonstration site was less than half the number at the Comparison site. Large volumes of new intermediate-level services were delivered. At the Demonstration site, children treated in intermediate residential settings spent, on average, almost 4 months in those facilities. For children treated in intermediate nonresidential settings, the average number of service encounters exceeded 60. Services designed to coordinate and facilitate treatment were used quite frequently, as well. Children received an average of 20 case management services. On average, treatment teams met approximately 3 times to discuss cases for which they were responsible.

Changes in cost-sharing alone[8] might lead one to predict that the

---

[7]The term "service encounter" denotes a day on which a service of a given type was received (see Chapter 2).

[8]Deductibles and copayments were waived at the Demonstration site.

Table 5.8. Mean Number of Services Received[a]

Period	Hospital (days)	RTC (days)	Intermediate residential (days)	Intermediate nonresidential (visits)	Outpatient (visits)	Assessment and evaluation	Case management (visits)	Treatment team (meetings)
Demonstration site								
Fiscal year								
1988	35.4	116.5	NA	NA	6.1	1.4	NA	NA
1989	34.8	137.3	NA	NA	6.0	1.4	NA	NA
1990				Transition period				
1991	33.8	59.2	78.9	38.8	14.0	1.5	6.1	2.0
1992	30.0	59.0	88.5	46.2	16.5	1.6	14.2	2.8
1993	24.9	51.8	85.5	46.8	18.4	2.0	24.5	2.0
Demonstration period	36.5	63.5	115.9	60.3	25.8	2.0	19.1	2.7
Comparison site								
Fiscal year								
1988	43.9	204.5	NA	NA	7.0	1.4	NA	NA
1989	44.3	186.8	NA	NA	6.7	1.4	NA	NA
1990	39.1	181.1	NA	NA	6.7	1.5	NA	NA
1991	32.1	134.5	NA	NA	7.5	1.7	NA	NA
1992	24.7	109.2	NA	NA	6.8	1.6	NA	NA
1993	31.0	96.7	NA	NA	6.5	1.7	NA	NA
Demonstration period	33.3	140.8	NA	NA	8.9	1.8	NA	NA

[a]These data describe the treated population at the Demonstration and Comparison sites. The Demonstration period is the combined fiscal years 1991–1993. The number of children for each entry is the same as that in the corresponding entry in Table 5.4. Each entry indicates the average number of services received. For example, the 152 children who were hospitalized at the Demonstration site in fiscal year 1988 spent an average of 35.4 days in the hospital.

volume of services delivered would increase, and there was such an increase. Table 5.8 also shows that outpatient visits in a given year more than doubled. In fiscal year 1991, for example, children at the Demonstration site who received outpatient services had 14 visits on average. Between fiscal year 1991 and fiscal year 1993, there was a trend toward increasing volume. By fiscal year 1993, the average number of outpatient visits (18.4) was over 3 times that for the Comparison site (6.5 visits). Another factor contributing to increased volume of services may have been the delayed implementation of the UR/M system. Because clinicians and reviewers apparently had insufficient data to consider the cost implications of utilization changes, cost-effectiveness could not be considered in treatment decisions as the UR/M Plan had stated it should be.

Between-site comparisons of days spent in hospitals were complicated. At the Demonstration site, the number of days hospitalized children spent in those facilities was lower in fiscal years 1991, 1992, and 1993 than prior to the Demonstration period. This comparison suggests that the volume of hospitalization at the Demonstration site decreased.[9] However, comparison for the entire Demonstration period across sites suggests that children hospitalized at the Demonstration site spent more time in the hospital than did children hospitalized under the traditional CHAMPUS care at the Comparison site. Children admitted to a hospital at the Demonstration site during the Demonstration period spend 3.2 more days in those facilities (36.5 days) than did children hospitalized at the Comparison site (33.3 days). Yearly data put the between-site comparison in a historical context and reveal trends over time, showing a steady reduction in volume of hospitalization at both sites. In addition, the difference in use between the two sites narrowed considerably. In fiscal year 1988, average use was over 1 week longer at the Comparison site, but by fiscal year 1992, the average was actually lower at the Comparison site than at the Demonstration site. During fiscal year 1993, however, the trend reversed at the Comparison site. In sum, the number of days children at the Demonstration site spent in hospitals fell, relative to historical levels, but not relative to children at the Comparison site.

[9]The number for the Demonstration period as a whole (36.5) exceeds that for fiscal year 1988 and fiscal year 1989. This does not indicate, however, that the volume of hospitalization increased, because the numbers are not comparable. Data for the Demonstration period pools not only the experiences of children treated in different years but also treatment a given child received in different years. A child, for example, might be hospitalized for 10 days in each year, contributing only 10 days to the yearly average but 30 days to the average for the entire period. The average for the Demonstration period is larger *not* because the child spent more time in the hospital, but because the window of relevant time is wider. (If children are hospitalized in only one year, there is no confusion: The average of the years equals the average for the Demonstration period.)

Table 5.9. Mean Length of Stay for Residential Admissions[a]

Period	Demonstration site			Comparison site	
	Hospital	RTC	Intermediate residential	Hospital	RTC
Fiscal year					
1988	35.34	181.35	NA	43.60	392.76
	(148)	(17)		(169)	(33)
1989	31.63	176.25	NA	47.23	371.26
	(187)	(12)		(194)	(23)
1990		Transition period		34.94	214.44
				(215)	(36)
1991	25.29	34.64	33.17	29.68	116.59
	(228)	(42)	(277)	(246)	(32)
1992	24.71	52.88	24.34	24.07	145.79
	(254)	(24)	(633)	(99)	(19)
1993	19.41	46.50	20.32	29.20	117.44
	(200)	(8)	(827)	(105)	(23)
Demonstration period	23.75	41.41	23.70	28.19	145.99
	(630)	(69)	(1533)	(420)	(67)

[a]These data describe the treated population at the Demonstration and Comparison sites. The figures for each time period pertain to admissions beginning in that period. The Demonstration-period admissions include those beginning between October 1, 1990, and June 1, 1993. Each entry indicates the average length of stay in days (and, in parentheses, the number of children admitted). For example, a hospital admission in fiscal year 1988 at the Demonstration site led to an average stay of 35.34 days, and a total of 148 children were admitted during that period.

Further analyses were conducted to better understand between-site differences in the use of hospitalization. A given number of days spent in the hospital may involve only one or more than one stay in the hospital; that is, children may be hospitalized once for a long period of time or repeatedly for short periods of time. Thus, the lengths of stays and number of admissions to hospitals and RTCs were examined.

Table 5.9 presents the mean LOS for admissions to hospitals, RTCs, and intermediate residential services at the Demonstration site.[10] Although differences between sites existed prior to the Demonstration, the Demonstration's effect on mean LOS is noticeable. Admissions during the Demonstration period led to LOS less than half as long in the Fort Bragg catchment area prior to the Demonstration. Yearly data show significant

[10]The figures for the Demonstration period as a whole are based on a somewhat different pool of children. Because of concerns that the data would not fully capture experiences of children still in a residential setting at the end of the period for which data were available, any admissions that did not begin before June 1, 1993, were omitted from the analysis. The contribution of fiscal year 1993, therefore, was reduced. Figures for fiscal year 1992, however, include all admissions.

reductions at the Comparison site as well, but they were not as great as those at the Demonstration site. RTC LOSs prior to Demonstration start-up at the Comparison site were double those at Fort Bragg. By the end of the Demonstration period, they were 3 times those at the Demonstration site.

Again, the issue of LOS extending across fiscal years is important. Because LOS is longer for RTCs than for hospitalization, the likelihood that an RTC stay will extend across fiscal years is greater. Also, RTC use was much higher in fiscal year 1991, so that its contribution is greater than in other years in determining the average for the period as a whole. Thus, the average hospital LOS for the Demonstration period is much nearer an average of the yearly LOSs than is the Demonstration-period average LOS for RTCs. Bearing this in mind, reduction in LOS does appear to explain the reduced number of days hospitalized children spent in the hospital. In fact, one would have expected an even greater decrease, since LOS was 3 times longer at the Comparison site initially. The only explanation is that children at the Demonstration site were hospitalized more frequently. In particular, children at the Demonstration site were more likely to return to the hospital. Table 5.10 shows the number of times a child who was hospitalized at least once was hospitalized. At the Demonstration site, repeat admissions were more likely; the average number of admissions was higher, and almost one third of those hospitalized during the Demonstration period were hospitalized more than once. These figures are more than double those for the Comparison site. Particularly noteworthy is the

Table 5.10. Number of Residential Admissions among Children Receiving Treatment in a Given Setting (Demonstration Period Only)[a]

Setting and site	Number of children	Distribution of number of admissions			Mean
		1	2	≥3	
Hospital					
Demonstration	432	70.6%	18.5%	10.9%	1.46
Comparison	359	85.5%	12.3%	2.2%	1.17
Residential treatment center					
Demonstration	54	25.9%	20.4%	3.7%	1.28
Comparison	64	96.9%	1.6%	1.5%	1.05
Intermediate residential					
Demonstration only	308	37.0%	13.6%	49.4%	4.97

[a]These data describe the treated population at the Demonstration and Comparison sites. The Demonstration period is the combined fiscal years 1991–1993. The entries in each row indicate the frequency distribution of the number of admissions to that setting and, in the last column, the mean number of admissions. Of children hospitalized at the Demonstration site, for example, 70.6% were admitted only once, and the mean number of admissions was 1.46.

likelihood of being hospitalized 3 or more times; this figure for the Demonstration site is nearly 5 times that for the Comparison site.

Data for the RTCs and intermediate residential services demonstrate a similar pattern. Children at the Demonstration site admitted to a given service at some point were much more likely than children at the Comparison site to be admitted again. Nearly half the children (49.4%) in intermediate residential care at the Demonstration site experienced 3 or more admissions to these facilities. It is worth noting, however, that these readmissions may not carry the negative connotation generally associated with repeated hospitalization. At the Demonstration site, children may move in and out of intermediate residential services in a planned fashion; this pattern may reflect the goals of the continuum of care.

This discussion of residential services has shown that a child treated at the Demonstration site was less likely to enter a hospital or an RTC than a child at the Comparison site. Upon entering such a facility, his or her stay was likely to be significantly shorter. The total time the child spent in such a facility during a given year, however, was inflated to some extent by the fact that he or she was more likely to return to that level of treatment at some point.

The discussion of whether the volume of hospitalization and other out-of-home treatment was lower at the Demonstration site thus far has been from the perspective of a child in the service system. At the Demonstration site, the child's chance of being hospitalized was lower. The perspective of the system administrator, however, is different. If one is interested, for instance, in whether the number of hospital beds should be decreased, the key piece of information is not the likelihood that a typical treated child will be placed in a hospital, but rather how many children are placed in a hospital and how many days those children spend in a hospital. From this perspective, it is clear that the Demonstration led to greater use of hospitalization, not less. Table 5.11 lists the number of children in residential or out-of-home placements. During the Demonstration period, a total of 501 children at the Demonstration site spent some time in a hospital. This number is considerably higher than that for the Comparison site (396). During the Demonstration period, 70 children at the Demonstration site compared to 91 children at the Comparison site were admitted to an RTC.

Further insight was gained by calculating the number of days children spent out of the home (see Table 5.12). Children at the Demonstration site spent a total of 22,745 days in hospitals or RTCs. This number is much lower than that for the Comparison site (25,999 days) and corresponds with the shorter LOS at the Demonstration site, as presented above. Combined with the fact that by fiscal year 1993 the yearly numbers had

Table 5.11. Number of Children in Out-of-Home Placements[a]

Period	Demonstration site			Comparison site	
	Hospital	RTC	Intermediate residential	Hospital	RTC
Fiscal year					
1988	152	19	NA	172	57
1989	176	18	NA	185	55
1990			Transition period	212	61
1991	197	45	87	236	50
1992	238	25	176	103	30
1993	181	6	200	99	29
Demonstration period	501	70	341	396	91

[a]These data describe the treated population at the Demonstration and Comparison sites. The Demonstration period is the combined fiscal years 1991–1993.

dropped to levels below those for years prior to the start of the Demonstration, it could have been concluded that the Demonstration reduced the use of out-of-home placements. However, when intermediate residential services at the Demonstration site are considered, the use of out-of-home placements must be reassessed. Children at the Demonstration site spent 62,281 days out of home. The reduction in the number of children placed in hospitals and RTCs and the time children spent in those facilities was offset by the use of intermediate residential care. The implications of this finding warrant further study; intermediate residential settings are designed to be less restrictive than hospitals or RTCs, and an offset in the use of these more restrictive services may be appropriate.

Distribution of Services over Time

An important dimension of utilization involves the timing of services received (i.e., the interval between services and the duration of treatment itself). Mental health services are consumed in "bundles" (Fowler, Keeler, & Keesey, 1981), and a convenient way of clustering service utilization measures is in episodes of treatment (Hornbrook, Hurtado, & Johnson, 1985). A frequent convention is to treat the passage of 8 weeks or more between services as ending one episode and beginning a new episode (Goldman, Scheffler, & Cheadle, 1987; Haas-Wilson, Cheadle, & Scheffler, 1989; Kessler, Steinwachs, & Hankin, 1980; Wells, Keeler, & Manning, 1990). The following discussion describes the episodes of care children experienced and the length of time they remained in treatment.

Any services received by the same child within an 8-week span are defined as falling into the same episode. In other words, a meaningful gap

Table 5.12. Days Out of the Home[a]

Period	Demonstration site					Comparison site		
	Hospital	RTC	Hospital + RTC	Intermediate residential	Total	Hospital	RTC	Total
Fiscal year								
1988	5,386	2,214	7,600	NA	7,600	7,551	11,654	19,205
1989	6,123	2,472	8,595	NA	8,595	8,213	10,272	18,485
1990			Transition period			8,294	11,045	19,339
1991	6,652	2,662	9,314	6,861	16,175	7,565	6,723	14,288
1992	7,132	1,474	8,606	15,572	24,178	2,540	3,275	5,815
1993	4,509	311	4,820	17,103	21,923	3,072	2,805	5,877
Demonstration period	18,298	4,447	22,745	39,536	62,281	13,186	12,813	25,999

[a]These data describe the treated population at the Comparison and Demonstration sites. The Demonstration period is the combined fiscal years 1991–1993.

Table 5.13. Nature of Episodes:
Episodes Beginning within the First Year of Treatment[a]

Period	Distribution of number of episodes				Mean number of episodes	Median episode (days)
	1	2	3	≥4		
Demonstration site						
Fiscal year						
1988 (N = 706)	73.1%	22.9%	3.5%	0.4%	1.3	31.0
1989 (N = 782)	77.2%	18.7%	3.5%	0.6%	1.3	32.0
1990			Transition period			
1991 (N = 2010)	67.2%	26.7%	5.4%	0.6%	1.4	87.0
1992 (N = 1641)	72.3%	24.0%	3.4%	0.3%	1.3	95.0
1993 (N = 1693)	79.4%	17.2%	2.9%	0.5%	1.2	89.0
Demonstration period (N = 4102)	69.9%	25.0%	4.5%	0.6%	1.4	93.0
Comparison site						
Fiscal year						
1988 (N = 727)	71.4%	20.9%	5.4%	2.3%	1.39	32.5
1989 (N = 797)	77.8%	17.3%	3.8%	1.1%	1.28	30.0
1990 (N = 775)	76.6%	18.1%	4.9%	0.9%	1.31	26.0
1991 (N = 819)	78.3%	18.8%	2.4%	0.5%	1.25	22.0
1992 (N = 620)	77.7%	17.3%	4.2%	0.8%	1.28	15.0
1993 (N = 738)	84.3%	13.3%	2.3%	0.1%	1.18	18.0
Demonstration period (N = 1601)	77.7%	18.2%	3.5%	0.6%	1.27	19.0

[a]These data describe the treated population at the Demonstration and Comparison sites. The figures for each time period pertain to children entering treatment in that period. The Demonstration period includes children entering treatment between October 1, 1990, and June 1, 1993. The entries in each row indicate the frequency distribution of the number of episodes occurring within the first year of treatment and, in the last two columns, the mean number of episodes and the median length of those episodes. For example, of children treated at the Demonstration site in fiscal year 1988, 73.1% had 1 episode of treatment; these children averaged 1.3 episodes of treatment, with a median episode length of 31 days.

in service use occurs when 8 weeks pass without the child's receiving any services. Table 5.13 presents basic descriptive information on the episodes of service use for the 365 days following the start of treatment.[11] It presents a percentage distribution of the number of episodes children experienced during the first year, the mean number of episodes, and the median length of those episodes. The sites were very similar prior to the Demonstration period; the mean number of episodes and the median length of episodes were nearly identical. The proportion of children at the Demonstration site

[11]More accurately, these figures describe the 365 days following the date on which records for the child appeared in the database. As discussed above, these data capture only services received in the three catchment areas. Thus, children may have received services prior to the time they appeared in our records.

who experienced only one episode in their first year of treatment fell somewhat (from 73.1% in fiscal year 1988 to 67.2% in fiscal year 1991). The proportion of children at the Comparison site who experienced only one episode of treatment in their first year of services increased in fiscal year 1993, perhaps because data for that year were truncated. Following a decrease in fiscal year 1992, this increase appears to reflect genuine changes in the system of care at the Comparison site.

In summary, the variation in the number of episodes was rather small. However, the median episode length for the Demonstration period tripled at the Demonstration site to nearly 3 months, indicating that children remained in treatment longer. This trend was verified by determining whether a child was in an episode of treatment 90, 180, and 365 days after first receiving services. Table 5.14 shows that for the pre-Demonstration years, the sites were comparable. After 180 days, fewer than 20% of children were still in an episode of service use. Figures for the Demonstration period, however, reveal striking differences between the sites. Children at the Demonstration site were much more likely to be still in care 90, 180, and 365 days after first receiving services. Nearly five eights of the children treated at the Demonstration site were still in an episode of care after 90 days, more than twice the rate for the Comparison site (21.8%). This difference persisted as children were followed for longer periods of time; at 180 days, 40.6% of the children at the Demonstration site were receiving care, compared to only 12.9% at the Comparison site.

It is clear that the Demonstration had a profound impact on the timing of services. The length of episodes of service increased dramatically, and children remained in treatment for significantly longer periods of time.

Continuity of Treatment

The discussion to this point has focused on whether a child received treatment and the type and volume of services received. It has also considered the timing of services received. Another aspect of service use, however, is the way in which services are ordered over time and how they fit together (i.e., continuity of care). The term *continuity* refers to coordination of services within the delivery system such that clients are able to move to and from settings without interruption (Bachrach, 1981). A principal concern is whether individuals who receive care in a residential setting have contact with the mental health system after discharge and, if they do, the setting and the time elapsed before contact occurs (Brown et al., 1994). Continuity of care is particularly pertinent to any analysis of a continuum of care, which is designed to "wrap" services around individuals so that

Table 5.14. Treatment Status after 90, 180, and 365 Days[a]

Period	90 Days			180 Days			365 Days		
	Not in treatment	In first episode	In second or later episode	Not in treatment	In first episode	In second or later episode	Not in treatment	In first episode	In second or later episode
Demonstration site									
Fiscal year									
1988 (N = 706)	72.1%	26.1%	1.8%	83.7%	11.2%	5.1%	90.7%	2.5%	6.8%
1989 (N = 782)	71.2%	26.9%	1.9%	83.6%	11.5%	4.8%	92.3%	3.5%	4.2%
1990									
Transition period									
1991 (N = 2010)	44.4%	53.1%	2.5%	60.8%	32.5%	6.7%	71.4%	15.4%	13.1%
1992 (N = 1641)	42.4%	55.7%	2.0%	59.7%	34.3%	6.1%	73.7%	15.8%	10.5%
1993 (N = 1693)	42.2%	56.2%	1.7%	59.2%	35.3%	5.5%	72.3%	19.1%	8.7%
Demonstration period (N = 4102)	42.8%	55.1%	2.1%	59.4%	34.3%	6.3%	72.4%	16.0%	11.6%
Comparison site									
Fiscal year									
1988 (N = 727)	72.5%	25.4%	2.1%	81.3%	13.1%	5.6%	88.7%	4.7%	5.6%
1989 (N = 797)	74.5%	23.1%	2.4%	82.9%	11.9%	5.2%	89.7%	3.9%	6.4%
1990 (N = 775)	78.8%	19.7%	1.4%	88.0%	8.1%	3.8%	91.1%	3.5%	5.4%
1991 (N = 819)	75.8%	21.4%	2.8%	87.4%	8.9%	3.7%	94.1%	1.8%	4.1%
1992 (N = 620)	79.7%	18.9%	1.5%	86.9%	8.7%	4.4%	94.0%	1.9%	4.1%
1993 (N = 738)	83.1%	15.9%	1.1%	88.5%	6.7%	4.9%	96.3%	0.6%	3.1%
Demonstration period (N = 1601)	78.2%	19.7%	2.1%	87.1%	8.7%	4.2%	94.3%	1.7%	3.9%

[a]These data describe the treated population at the Demonstration and Comparison sites. The percentages for each time period pertain to children entering treatment in that period. The Demonstration period includes children entering treatment between October 1, 1990, and June 1, 1993. The table indicates the status of treated children at 90, 180, 365 days after beginning treatment as being in one of three categories: not in treatment, in their first episode of service utilization, or in a second or later episode. For example, of the children who entered treatment in fiscal year 1988 at the Demonstration site, 72.1% were no longer in treatment after 90 days.

transitions between levels of care[12] are seamless. A distinguishing feature of the Demonstration is that it provided intermediate services and services (e.g., case management) designed to smooth the transition to less restrictive settings. The following discussion considers whether continuity (i.e., the transition to less restrictive settings) was actually better at the Demonstration site.

The preceding discussion of episodes shed some light on continuity of care. Children receiving care with less continuity would be more likely to have a disruption in their care (i.e., to have more episodes) than children treated for a similar period of time in a continuum. Such as comparison can be made using the data in Table 5.14. Prior to the Demonstration period (i.e., in fiscal year 1988), roughly 70% of children still in treatment after 180 days were still in their first episode at both sites.[13] These children had no disruptions of treatment of more than 8 weeks in length. For the Demonstration period, however, this figure rose to 84.5%. This finding suggests that children received care with greater continuity.

The foregoing discussion of episodes and disruptions in service use was based on the dates on which services were received; the types of services and the order in which they were received were not considered. A related aspect of the continuity of care, however, involves the way in which services fit together. One measure of continuity is the receipt of follow-up care in the community after discharge from a hospital. Table 5.15 describes the first service children received within 30 days of discharge from a hospital or an RTC. It can be seen that at the Demonstration site, children were much more likely to receive care within 30 days and to receive it in a less restrictive setting. Five of six clients at the Demonstration site received a less restrictive service within 30 days, fewer than 7% received no services, and only 8.2% returned to a hospital or RTC. In comparison, over 50% of the children discharged at the Comparison site received no follow-up service, and almost 14% returned to a hospital or RTC.

Intermediate services at the Demonstration site were designed to provide a transition from more to less restrictive settings, and they appear to have functioned as intended. Of the children at the Demonstration site who received care within the first 30 days of discharge, the majority received care that was not available under CHAMPUS; they were served

---

[12]The Demonstration developers and advocates of the continuum of care specifically prefer transitions to be from most to least restrictive rather than vice versa. The restrictiveness issue was addressed above.

[13]The calculation for the Fort Bragg catchment area for fiscal year 1988 equals the conditional probability, p (Children in first episode after 180 days/Children still in treatment after 180 days), which equals 11.2%/(11.2% + 5.1%) = 68.7%.

Table 5.15. Transitions from Hospital or Residential Treatment Center: First Service Received within 30 Days of Discharge[a]

Period	First service received within 30 days						
	No service received	Hospital/ RTC	Intermediate residential	Intermediate nonresidential	Case management treatment team	Outpatient	Other
Demonstration site							
Fiscal year							
1988 (N = 165)	52.7%	10.3%	NA	NA	NA	30.3%	6.7%
1989 (N = 199)	55.3%	11.6%	NA	NA	NA	31.7%	1.5%
1990				Transition period			
1991 (N = 270)	9.6%	12.6%	11.5%	10.7%	24.4%	29.6%	0.0%
1992 (N = 278)	5.4%	6.8%	17.3%	13.7%	44.6%	12.2%	0.0%
1993 (N = 208)	3.4%	1.9%	14.4%	12.5%	59.1%	8.7%	0.0%
Demonstration period (N = 699)	6.9%	8.2%	14.0%	11.9%	40.2%	18.3%	0.0%
Comparison site							
Fiscal year							
1988 (N = 202)	59.9%	6.9%	NA	NA	NA	32.7%	0.5%
1989 (N = 217)	54.8%	8.3%	NA	NA	NA	35.9%	0.9%
1990 (N = 251)	55.8%	9.6%	NA	NA	NA	32.3%	2.4%
1991 (N = 278)	53.2%	14.0%	NA	NA	NA	31.7%	0.8%
1992 (N = 118)	50.9%	12.7%	NA	NA	NA	35.6%	0.9%
1993 (N = 128)	58.6%	10.9%	NA	NA	NA	30.5%	0.0%
Demonstration period (N = 487)	52.8%	13.6%	NA	NA	NA	32.9%	0.8%

[a]These data describe the treated population at the Demonstration and Comparison sites. The Demonstration period includes discharges from hospitals or RTCs that occurred between October 1, 1990, and June 1, 1993. The unit of observation is the discharge; some patients contribute more than one unit. The percentages indicate the first service received within 30 days by children who were discharged. For example, of the children discharged in fiscal year 1988 at the Demonstration site, 52.7% received no service within 30 days.

in an intermediate setting, received case management, or had a treatment team meeting.

In summary, the Demonstration site delivered greater continuity of care. Children leaving the hospital did not leave the system. Rather, they received services (either direct or of a case management nature) within 30 days.

Were Children Treated Differently or Were Different Children Treated?

The differences in service utilization documented thus far suggest that moving a child from one site to the other would alter the care he or she received. Before drawing this conclusion, however, the Project considered alternative explanations. The tables presented thus far attempted to describe the treatment that a "typical" child received at each site, and comparisons between sites assumed that the typical child was comparable across sites. In other words, the typical child at the Comparison site, were he or she moved across sites, would have received the services that the typical child at the Demonstration site received. Given the dramatic increase in access to services at the Demonstration site, however, this assumption was a fairly strong one. It implied that the large changes in access that occurred at the Demonstration site had no effect on the mix of children treated, that the "new" children who entered the system did not differ systematically from those already receiving services. If this assumption was incorrect, data presented thus far may reveal only that different children were treated differently at the sites. To test whether the assumption about case mix was warranted, the Evaluation Sample was used to examine differences in the treatment that children of comparable severity at Wave 1[14] received at different sites.

Table 5.16 describes the most restrictive service that children in the Evaluation Sample received between Waves 1 and 2 of data collection. The bottom row of the table presents figures for the Evaluation Sample as a whole. As noted above, children at the Demonstration site were far less likely to be hospitalized or to receive outpatient care only. Slightly more than 1 in 5 (22.3%) received intermediate services as their most restrictive service.[15]

---

[14]The severity of the child's overall mental health status was quantified as a z-weighted average of total P-CAS psychopathology and overall CAFAS impairment in functioning. Severity, then, encompassed symptoms and functioning in one overall index.

[15]Children in the Evaluation Sample received more restrictive services as a group, a reflection of sampling methodology (see Chapter 2).

Table 5.16. Comparison of Most Restrictive Service Received by Severity[a]

Severity and site	Number of children	Most restrictive service by severity					
		Hospitalization	RTC	Intermediate residential	Intermediate nonresidential	Outpatient
Least severe						
Demonstration	151	3.3%	1.3%	4.0%	9.3%	82.1%
Comparison	93	8.6%	0.0%	NA	NA	91.4%
Moderately severe						
Demonstration	279	14.7%	0.0%	4.7%	20.1%	60.6%
Comparison	210	22.4%	0.0%	NA	NA	77.6%
Most severe						
Demonstration	143	41.3%	0.0%	10.5%	16.8%	31.5%
Comparison	102	56.9%	3.9%	NA	NA	39.2%
Evaluation sample total						
Demonstration	573	18.3%	0.4%	5.9%	16.4%	59.0%
Comparison	405	27.9%	1.0%	NA	NA	71.1%

[a]These data describe the experiences of the Evaluation Sample between 1 and 2. The entries in each row indicate the distribution across service types for children of a given level of severity at each site. For example, 3.3% of children of least severity at the Demonstration site were hospitalized between waves 1 and 2. The number of choices differs by site, so standard tests of joint significance in contingency tables are inappropriate. The zeros in the intermediate columns occur not by chance, but must equal zero. Separate significance tests were conducted for the likelihood of hospitalization or outpatient therapy, and differed by site.

Table 5.16 also presents the most restrictive service for the least to most severely impaired children.[16] Regardless of the child's level of severity, children at the Demonstration site were less likely to be hospitalized. This difference is especially large in the least severe cases, among whom a child at the Comparison site was 2.5 times more likely to be hospitalized than a similarly impaired child at the Demonstration site. Likewise, across all three severity groups, children at the Comparison site were far more likely to have only outpatient care as their most "restrictive" service, since no intermediate services were available.

The documented differences in service utilization, therefore, do not appear to be a result of different children being treated. Instead, comparable children were treated differently. It does appear that if a child were moved from the Comparison site to the Demonstration site, he or she would have received different services.

SATISFACTION WITH TREATMENT

This section considers the perspectives of consumers. Parents and children were asked to rate their satisfaction with several dimensions of the various services they received. Parents' and children's satisfaction with mental health services received in the previous 6 months was assessed at Waves 2 and 3. The Satisfaction Scales, developed for the Project, include nine separate modules, each with an adolescent and a parent version. Each module assesses satisfaction with a different type of service (e.g., outpatient, case management, after-school, or therapeutic home services). Findings from the intake and assessment module were reported in Chapter 4. This chapter includes findings about treatment components.

Parent ratings of satisfaction with services were available from a wide range of treatment levels categorized as inpatient hospitalization or RTC care, intermediate residential or nonresidential services, and outpatient services. While all three of these levels of services were available at the Demonstration site, only inpatient/RTC and outpatient care were available at the Comparison site. Consequently, between-site comparisons of satisfaction are restricted to those services that are common to both sites. The dimensions on which satisfaction with services was assessed and compared included: (1) access and convenience, (2) treatment provided to the child, (3) services to parents, (4) services to families, (5) coordination of

[16]Severity was defined as a composite score consisting of standardized symptom and level of functioning scores.

services, (6) relationship with the child's therapist, (7) financial charges, (8) discharge and transition planning, and (9) global satisfaction.

Comparison across Sites for Traditional CHAMPUS Services[17]

Tables 5.17–5.20 present between-site comparisons for outpatient and inpatient/RTC services reported by parents and adolescents. Note that the scores in these tables are standardized for each of the four groups and are not comparable across these four tables. However, Table 5.21 and the accompanying text address global satisfaction with treatment across sites.

Outpatient Services

In Table 5.17, parents' satisfaction with outpatient services their children received at the Demonstration and Comparison sites is examined. In each of the areas of satisfaction, parents at the Demonstration site reported being significantly more satisfied with services their children received than did the parents at the Comparison site. For every component, parents at the Comparison site reported satisfaction levels below the pooled mean, while parents at the Demonstrate site reported higher than average satisfaction.

Table 5.18 shows the between-site differences in satisfaction as reported by adolescents who received outpatient services. Significant differences were found in two of the eight areas of satisfaction, and differences in three other areas approached significance. Adolescents at the Demonstration site reported being significantly more satisfied with the access to and convenience of services and their relationships with their therapists.

Inpatient/RTC Services

Table 5.19 presents the comparison of parents' reports of satisfaction with services received by their children for inpatient/RTC settings between the Demonstration and Comparison sites. Statistically significant differences in levels of satisfaction were found for only two of the inpatient/RTC components of satisfaction. Parents at the Demonstration site reported significantly higher satisfaction with access to and convenience of inpatient/RTC services and the financial charges associated with those

---

[17]For these analyses, satisfaction data collected at Waves 2 and 3 were combined in order to provide the most comprehensive examination of consumer reports. Because it was possible for respondents to complete multiple modules, one scale per respondent was randomly selected to be included in these analyses.

Table 5.17. Follow-Up Comparisons:
Parents' Satisfaction with Outpatient Services

Component of satisfaction	Demonstration site (D)			Comparison site (C)			D–C ES	p(F)[b]
	Mean[a]	SD	N	Mean[a]	SD	N		
Access and convenience	0.14[c]	0.71	401	−0.19	0.81	297	0.44	<0.01
Child's treatment	0.20[c]	0.78	374	−0.25	0.91	269	0.54	<0.01
Parent services	0.23[c]	0.85	362	−0.21	0.90	274	0.51	<0.01
Family services	0.31[c]	0.86	336	−0.26	0.85	239	0.66	<0.01
Coordination of services	0.18[c]	0.93	139	−0.28	1.04	91	0.47	<0.01
Relationship with therapist	0.19[c]	0.69	395	−0.25	0.78	276	0.60	<0.01
Financial charges	0.30[c]	0.57	321	−0.39	0.86	233	1.00	<0.01
Discharge/transition planning	0.25[c]	0.82	127	−0.18	0.83	122	0.54	<0.01
Global satisfaction	0.23[c]	0.78	351	−0.26	0.98	239	0.57	<0.01

[a]Means reflect mean subscale scores generated using standardized item scores with a mean of 0. Items were standarized on a sample of pooled sites, and across follow-up waves, limited to one Satisfaction Scale per respondent. More positive scores indicate greater satisfaction. These standardized scores were calculated independently for each group of respondents by type of service. Therefore, scores in Tables 5.17–5.20 cannot be compared.

[b]p(F)<0.01 defined statistical significance for these comparisons. The assumption of independence necessary for these analyses was threatened by the sample of parents reporting about services provided by a smaller number of providers. In an effort to counter this threat, it was determined a priori to use the more conservative p-value of ≤0.01 to indicate significance.

[c]There was a statistically significant difference between the Demonstration and Comparison site means.

Table 5.18. Follow-Up Comparisons:
Adolescents' Satisfaction with Outpatient Services

Component of satisfaction	Demonstration site (D)			Comparison site (C)			D–C ES	p(F)[b]
	Mean[a]	SD	N	Mean[a]	SD	N		
Access and convenience	0.11[c]	0.65	151	−0.12	0.74	142	0.33	<0.01
Child's treatment	0.10	0.73	168	−0.08	0.86	149	0.23	0.04
Parent services	−0.04	0.96	153	0.04	1.04	140	−0.08	0.53
Family services	0.00	0.96	153	0.01	1.05	141	−0.01	0.93
Coordination of services	−0.06	0.97	98	0.06	1.03	94	−0.12	0.43
Relationship with therapist	0.11[c]	0.56	176	−0.13	0.66	155	0.39	<0.01
Discharge/transition planning	0.11	0.73	45	−0.22	0.76	48	0.44	0.04
Global satisfaction	0.12	0.75	114	−0.15	0.90	119	0.33	0.02

[a]–[c]See Table 5.17 footnotes.

Table 5.19. Follow-Up Comparisons:
Parents' Satisfaction with Inpatient/RTC Services

Component of satisfaction	Demonstration site (D)			Comparison site (C)			D–C ES	$p(F)^b$
	Mean^a	SD	N	Mean^a	SD	N		
Access and convenience	0.20^c	0.69	68	−0.13	0.74	89	0.46	<0.01
Child's treatment	−0.04	0.94	68	0.02	0.82	90	−0.07	0.65
Parent services	−0.08	1.02	67	0.09	0.83	89	−0.19	0.26
Family services	−0.05	1.00	65	0.10	0.89	85	−0.16	0.36
Relationship with therapist	−0.11	0.94	66	0.07	0.75	87	−0.22	0.20
Staff responsiveness	−0.13	0.95	64	0.13	0.80	86	−0.30	0.08
Financial charges	0.17^c	0.87	57	−0.20	0.81	82	0.45	0.01
Discharge/transition planning	0.14	0.93	60	−0.13	0.77	59	0.32	0.09
Global satisfaction	−0.05	0.98	59	0.16	0.86	58	−0.23	0.23

$^{a–c}$See Table 5.17 footnotes.

services than did parents at the Comparison site. Lack of differences in other inpatient/RTC areas may be explained by the difficulty inherent in persuading established residential services providers to alter their delivery of services. As noted above, the Demonstration site did not provide these services directly, but through contacts with area inpatient hospitals and RTCs. It is noteworthy that differences in satisfaction were found in areas more easily influenced by the Demonstration.

Adolescents' satisfaction with inpatient/RTC services is reported in Table 5.20. At the $p \leq 0.01$ level, no statistically significant differences were found between satisfaction reported by adolescents at the Demonstration and Comparison sites. However, it should be noted that the very small sample sizes likely constrained this analysis.[18]

Global Satisfaction with Treatment

For these analyses, data from Waves 2 and 3 were combined and one randomly selected scale per respondent was included. Subscale scores were calculated from raw items, each having a 4-point response set ranging from 1 ("very dissatisfied") to 4 ("very satisfied") in order to allow comparison of ratings between different treatment settings and respon-

[18]In order to achieve sufficient power (0.80) to detect an effect size of SD 0.25, each group had to include at least 375 respondents (Lipsey, 1990).

Table 5.20. Follow-Up Comparisons:
Adolescents' Satisfaction with Inpatient/RTC Services

Component of satisfaction	Demonstration site (D)			Comparison site (C)			D–C ES	$p(F)^b$
	Mean[a]	SD	N	Mean[a]	SD	N		
Access and convenience	0.07	0.64	13	0.12	0.74	23	−0.07	0.84
Child's treatment	−0.16	0.84	32	0.12	0.88	37	−0.33	0.18
Parent services	−0.22	0.96	33	0.20	1.01	36	−0.24	0.08
Family services	−0.26	1.01	16	0.18	0.98	23	−0.44	0.18
Coordination of services	−0.14	1.07	26	0.14	0.93	27	−0.28	0.31
Relationship with therapist	−0.06	0.72	35	0.04	0.74	54	−0.14	0.55
Staff responsiveness	−0.12	0.81	34	0.03	0.86	37	−0.18	0.43
Discharge/transition planning	−0.06	0.74	25	0.20	0.82	28	−0.33	0.23
Global satisfaction	−0.09	0.83	33	0.07	0.84	52	−0.19	0.38

[a-c]See Table 5.17 footnotes.

dent groups. As can be seen in Table 5.21, both parents and adolescents at the Demonstration site reported being more satisfied with outpatient services than did their counterparts at the Comparison site. However, no differences were found between reports of global satisfaction with inpatient/RTC services. These results are similar to those reported above, but reflect only the ratings on global satisfaction. Table 5.21 includes the means and standard deviations calculated from parents' and adolescents' reports of global satisfaction with intermediate-level services received at the Demonstration site. Mean scores for parents' satisfaction with intermediate services tended to be slightly higher than the middle of the range (2.5), with after-school and therapeutic home programs receiving the lowest satisfaction ratings.

In general, adolescents' mean scores for global satisfaction with intermediate services were also slightly higher than the middle of the range. Ratings for case management and group home services were both above the midpoint, while the others were slightly below it. On average, both parents and adolescents reported being satisfied with intermediate services they received. Adolescents reported slightly lower levels of satisfaction than parents. A trend emerged when services at the Demonstration site were rank-ordered according to respondent ratings of global satisfaction. In general, case management, outpatient, and group home services were rated highest. The exception to this trend was differential ranking for

Table 5.21. Follow-Up Comparisons:
Parents' and Adolescents' Satisfaction with Services

Component of satisfaction	Demonstration site (D)			Comparison site (C)			D–C ES	$p(F)^b$
	Mean[a]	SD	N	Mean[a]	SD	N		
			Parents					
Day treatment	3.45	0.66	47	—	—	—		—
Case management	3.34	0.79	108	—	—	—		—
Outpatient	3.33[c]	0.73	414	2.84	0.90	297	0.61	<0.01
Group home	3.18	0.70	25	—	—	—		—
In-home services	3.13	0.95	43	—	—	—		0.49
Inpatient/RTC	2.85	1.01	68	2.96	0.89	88	−0.12	—
After-school	2.78	1.11	13	—	—	—		—
Therapeutic home	2.76	1.09	26	—	—	—		—
			Adolescents					
Case management	3.30	0.84	23	—	—	—		—
Group home	3.22	0.65	13	—	—	—		—
Outpatient	3.21[c]	0.58	179	2.92	0.75	161	0.44	<0.01
In-home services	2.92	0.82	12	—	—	—		—
Therapeutic home	2.89	1.04	12	—	—	—		—
After-school	2.83	0.77	7	—	—	—		—
Inpatient/RTC	2.69	0.85	35	2.89	0.85	52	−0.24	0.27
Day treatment	2.61	0.85	17	—	—	—		—

[a]Scale: 1 ("very dissatisfied") to 4 ("very satisfied"). Means reflect mean scores on the 5-item global satisfaction subscale of the Satisfaction Scale corresponding to each service component. Subscale scores were calculated using raw item scores that were comparable across Satisfaction Scales. Means were generated on a sample of pooled sites, and across follow-up waves, limited to 1 Satisfaction Scale per respondent.
[b,c]See Table 5.17 footnotes.

day treatment services; parents' ratings resulted in a top ranking, while adolescents' ratings resulted in the lowest rank.

THE TREATMENT PROCESS AND SERVICE UTILIZATION: SUMMARY OF FINDINGS

Provision of a comprehensive and coordinated array of service options is a critical element of the Demonstration. Extensive examination in earlier reports (Heflinger, 1993; Bickman et al., 1993) revealed that the Demonstration's continuum of care was well implemented with sufficient quality to test the program model. At the Comparison site, however, services were limited to traditional outpatient services and residential services (inpatient hospitals and RTCs). Services at the Comparison site were not linked by formal case management, as they were at the Demonstration site.

When community experts were asked to rate mental health services for military dependents in their communities, they reported significantly greater adequacy and quality of the components of treatment at the Demonstration site. In addition, on items assessing service system performance regarding aspects of treatment, the Demonstration site received significantly more positive ratings.

The Demonstration had a dramatic effect on service utilization. Service use was examined by focusing on five dimensions: type, mix, volume, distribution over time, and continuity of services received. The program model of the Demonstration would predict that each of these dimensions would be affected greatly.

The *types* of services delivered changed: Intermediate services previously unavailable were used by large numbers of clients, and a layer of services (treatment team services and clinical case management) was used extensively to coordinate the other services. The *mix* of services also changed: Children moved toward the middle of the continuum of care; a child treated at the Demonstration site was less likely to receive care in a hospital or RTC, but was also less likely to receive only outpatient treatment. This shift in service mix conformed to the prescriptions of the program theory underlying the Demonstration. Children appeared to appropriately receive the newly available intermediate services; those who were hospitalized were far more likely to receive intermediate ("stepdown") services than clients who were not.

The *volume* of services was affected as well: The volume of the "new" intermediate services used was quite large. Clients receiving outpatient therapy had significantly more visits at the Demonstration site. Children at the Demonstration site spent more days in out-of-home placements. Children hospitalized or treated in RTCs, however, spent less time in those facilities at the Demonstration site.

The Demonstration also influenced the *timing* of services. Children at the Demonstration site were far more likely to remain in treatment and less likely to have experienced a significant interruption in their treatment. Improved *continuity* was also apparent in the way services "fit together": Upon leaving a hospital or RTC, children at the Demonstration site were far more likely to receive follow-up services in a less restrictive setting within 30 days.

It appears that differences in service utilization between sites were not simple manifestations of shifts in the mix of children treated. Comparisons of children in the Evaluation Sample who started services at a comparable level of severity confirmed earlier results; children at the Demonstration site received markedly different treatment.

The Demonstration site received significantly higher ratings of parent satisfaction with outpatient treatment in all components of satisfaction, while adolescents endorsed two of the eight areas more positively. Parents at the Demonstration site reported significantly higher satisfaction with two components of inpatient/RTC treatment: (1) access to inpatient/RTC services and (2) convenience and financial charges.

When only items reflecting global satisfaction were considered, two trends emerged. First, both parents and adolescents at the Demonstration site reported significantly higher satisfaction with outpatient services than did respondents at the Comparison site, while no statistically significant differences were reported for inpatient/RTC services. Second, in general, when services at the Demonstration site were rank-ordered according to respondent ratings, services were ranked similarly, for the most part, by parents and adolescents. In general, case management, outpatient, and group home services were rated highest; inpatient, after-school, and therapeutic home programs were rated lowest. The exception to this trend was the differential ranking for day treatment services. Parents' ratings resulted in the highest ranking, while adolescents' ratings resulted in the lowest.

SYSTEM QUALITY: APPROPRIATENESS

The concept of the quality of the treatment system is critical to the program model, which hypothesized that the major impact of the continuum of care would be on the provision of more appropriate services. The hypothesized clinical and cost superiority of the continuum is contingent on the appropriate assignment of children to different levels of care and on timely transitions between these levels. "Appropriateness" is the Project's term for describing the proximal outcome related to the processes of treatment planning and case management as shown in Figure 5.1.

As the program model indicates, more accurate diagnosis should lead to better treatment planning. A multidisciplinary and standardized treatment planning process should produce a treatment plan that fits the child's and family's needs better and is a better match to the child's problems. The availability of the full continuum of care services allows the child to receive the most appropriate services. Case management helps ensure that the child's treatment is monitored and that shifts in levels of care occur at appropriate times. Nothing in this conceptualization of the continuum of care implies that the actual therapy that is delivered is superior or that clinicians delivering this therapy are better therapists than those at the Comparison site.

The continuum at the Demonstration site is different from the services at the Comparison site in two significant ways: (1) the high quality of the service delivery *system* and (2) the availability of a *wide variety of services*. These services should match the child's needs better than those in the Comparison site. The logic model indicates that there are a number of elements that compose a quality system of care. Each of these elements is described below, and relevant data described earlier are reviewed.

Elements of Quality of a System of Care

Continuity

Continuity refers to the transitions from one service level to another and the absence of significant gaps in treatment. A high-quality system of care should be characterized by smooth and timely transitions between different levels of care. For example, a child leaving an intensive level of care should receive a less intensive service in a timely manner. Continuity was measured in two ways. First, the proportion of clients who received a less intensive service within 30 days of the occurrence of the last day of an episode of restrictive residential care (hospital or RTC) was examined. Second, the breaks or interruptions in service were delimited by examining the number and length of episodes of care.

There were dramatic differences between the Demonstration and Comparison sites in the way in which children made transitions from hospitals and RTCs to other levels of service. During the Demonstration period, over 93% of children at the Demonstration site received a service within the 30 days of discharge, compared to 47% of children at the Comparison site (Table 5.15). Moreover, it was more likely that the subsequent service was another hospital stay at the Comparison site than at the Demonstration site. Additionally, treatment episodes were substantially longer at the Demonstration site. Children stayed in treatment longer and there was a higher percentage of children still in their first episode after 90, 180, and 365 days.

It is clear from both these measures that there was greater continuity of care at the Demonstration site. Children were less likely to have a break in treatment. Continuity, as an indicator of the quality of the system of care, was far better at the Demonstration site than at the Comparison site.

Dropouts from Treatment

In general, a quality system of care should result in better communication between the family and the therapist. More specifically, the family and the therapist should evidence more agreement on length of treatment and when treatment should be terminated. Moreover, a better system of care should result in more children successfully completing treatment without premature termination. Treatment termination was studied two ways. First, parents were asked who initiated termination. This method assessed agreement between the therapist and the family from the parent's perspective. Second, for the entire population of children treated, the percentage of children who had only one outpatient visit was calculated. It was assumed that it was unlikely a single visit would result in resolution of a significant problem and that a significant problem existed if a diagnosis was warranted.

Parent's Perspective of Agreement Regarding Treatment Termination. In a better system of care, there should be more agreement between the clinician and the family to terminate services. At the Demonstration site, 64.7% of parents agreed with the clinician as to whether services should be continued or terminated. At the Comparison site, 53.6% of parents agreed with the therapist. Interestingly, especially given the longer lengths of service at the Demonstration site, fewer than 7% of parents there said they initiated termination of service, compared to 18.3% at the Comparison site.

Premature Termination of Treatment. To assess dropout rates for the entire treated population, the records of all children who received services at both sites were compared to the percentage of children who received only one outpatient visit. The dropout rate was more than 3 times as high at the Comparison site (24% compared to 7% at the Demonstration site).

These data are consistent with the conclusion that treatment was terminated at the Demonstration site more appropriately than at the Comparison site. The rate of single treatment sessions was much lower and parents were more in agreement with the therapist as to when to terminate treatment at the Demonstration site.

Restrictiveness of Care

A system that provides care at the least restrictive level, without adverse clinical effects, is seen as providing more appropriate care than one that relies on more restrictive services. To evaluate this aspect, service utilization data were examined to determine whether a greater proportion of children at the Demonstration site were treated in less restrictive environments. This evaluation was made for both the catchment populations and the Evaluation Sample, in which children could be matched on level of severity to help ensure that clinically comparable children were being compared.

Over the 3-year Demonstration period, only 8.6% of children at the Demonstration site received care in a hospital or RTC, compared to 15.7%

at the Comparison site (Table 5.5). This finding is not compromised by the inclusion of intermediate residential care, which accounted for an additional 2.4% of the children and brought the total at the Demonstration site for the Demonstration period to 11%.

This finding was duplicated when only the Evaluation Sample was considered. It was possible to match children on initial level of severity, and at every level children at the Comparison site were placed in a hospital or RTC at a higher rate than were children at the Demonstration site.

Individualized Care

A more appropriate system of care should match family and child needs with services. By offering a wide variety of service options, it is possible to provide more individualized care. Rather than fitting the child to the services, the services are "wrapped around" the child. Individualized care was assessed in two ways. First, at the population level and within the Evaluation Sample, a "service mix ratio" was calculated for each child. This ratio reflected the diversity of services received and was used as an index of the range of services actually received by the children in both systems. Second, the match between child and family needs was also examined from the parent's perspective, on the basis of data from the Satisfaction Scales.

Service Mix Ratio. Using the rationale that more severe children should receive a greater "mix" of services, both the Evaluation Sample and the treated population were examined. For the Evaluation Sample, one would expect that more severe children would receive more services of different types. The most severely impaired children (the 25% with the highest severity ratings) at the Demonstration site typically received from 2 to 3 different types of services, while children at the Comparison site received between 1 and 2.

In the treated-population analysis, because the Project had no measure of severity at the population level, the receipt of more-than-outpatient treatment was used as a proxy. As illustrated in Figure 5.2, children at the Demonstration site who received any services that were more-than-outpatient were more likely to receive a greater number of different types of services[19] than their counterparts at the Comparison site.

[19]The types of services used were hospital, RTC, intermediate residential, intermediate nonresidential, outpatient, and medical evaluation. Intermediate services were not available at the Comparison site, limiting the maximum number of service types received at the Comparison site to 4.

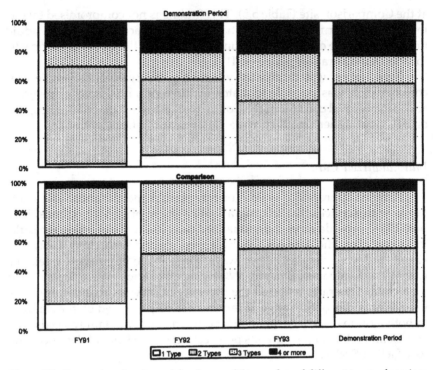

Figure 5.2. Comparison by site and fiscal year of the number of different types of services received.

Satisfaction with the Match between Service and Needs.   The match between child and family needs was examined from parents' and adolescents' perspectives on satisfaction with services received. Only data from the Satisfaction Scales for typical residential (inpatient/RTC) and outpatient services were used for this analysis, since only these services were available at both sites. Parents of children receiving outpatient treatment at the Demonstration site were significantly more satisfied with the match between their children's and families' needs (χ^2, $p \leq 0.01$), while no difference was found between sites according to adolescents' satisfaction reports. When residential services data were examined, adolescents at the Demonstration site were significantly more satisfied with the match between their own and their families' needs (χ^2, $p \leq 0.01$), while no difference was found between sites according to parents' reports. Hence, when there were significant differences in satisfaction with the match between needs and treatment received, the differences favored the Demonstration site.

Timeliness

A more appropriate system of care should place children in services as quickly as possible. The Demonstration site was required by contract to assess and begin treating children in a timely manner (see Chapter 4). The Comparison site had no such requirements. The Demonstration Management Information System provided data used to evaluate this criterion for the Demonstration site. For the Comparison site, the CHAMPUS data did not provide a separate designation for intake and assessment or screening. Thus, in order to compare the two systems of care, the Project assumed that the time between the first and second visit at the Comparison site was comparable to the time between the intake and assessment and the first clinical service at the Demonstration site. This assumption was based on clinicians' responses for the Quality Study, in which they indicated that the first visit usually served as an assessment visit. The Demonstration site outperformed the Comparison site in timeliness between assessment and treatment (17 days at the Demonstration site compared to 38 days at the Comparison site).

No utilization data were available regarding the time between a parent's request for services and delivery of the first service. However, data on client satisfaction presented in Chapter 4 indicated greater satisfaction at the Demonstration site with the time waiting for services.

Summary of Appropriateness

The Demonstration achieved the following objectives:

- Provided greater continuity of treatment.
- Had fewer dropouts from treatment.
- Appeared to place children in less restrictive, yet appropriate settings.
- Provided more individualized treatment.
- Delivered services in a more timely manner.

Thus, the Demonstration site provided the higher-quality system of care as presented in the program model.

6

Mental Health Outcomes

Questions central to the Outcome Study focused on whether children at the Demonstration site showed improvement in mental health outcome, whether such improvement was greater than that of children in more typical mental health services, and whether characteristics of children or families related to differences in outcome. These questions relate to the ultimate outcome areas of the program model labeled "Improved mental health outcomes" and "Quicker recovery" (Figure 6.1).

This chapter begins by explaining the Project's data structure and discussing children's response to treatment at the individual level. From there, changes in children's mental health status are presented in terms of diagnostic change and parents' opinions about their children's improvement. Key mental health outcome measures are described, followed by an analysis of change based on these outcome measures. Global change is explored with more precise analyses. Finally, specific hypotheses about subgroups expected to change within the continuum-of-care model are presented and tested.

INTRODUCTION TO MENTAL HEALTH OUTCOMES: WAVE-BY-SITE DATA COMPARISONS

An important step in comprehending the analyses that follow is understanding the wave-by-site organization of the Project's mental health outcome data. As discussed in Chapter 2, families participated in three waves of data collection. Wave 1 data were collected approximately at the time of intake into services, Wave 2 data approximately 6 months later, and Wave 3 data approximately 1 year following intake.

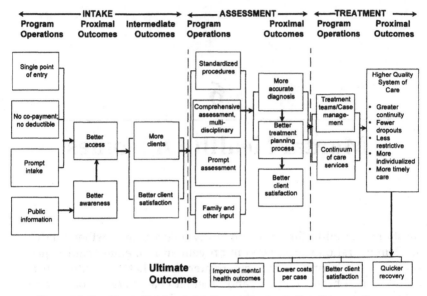

Figure 6.1. Fort Bragg Child and Adolescent Demonstration: Program theory.

Figure 6.2 shows mean scores for two mental health measurements by wave and site (Demonstration and Comparison). Figures 6.2–6.5 provide an overview of how children's mental health changed during the Evaluation.

For the total Evaluation Sample, the mean Child Behavior Checklist (CBCL) score was approximately 65 (in the clinical range) at Wave 1, and mean scores lowered (improved) at Waves 2 and 3. This pattern held for both the Demonstration site and the Comparison site; at both, mean scores dropped to well within the nonclinical range. This improvement is consistent with the meta-analysis of Lipsey and Wilson (1993), which found positive outcomes for many psychological, educational, and behavioral treatments. Scores on the child-reported Youth Self-Report (YSR) at both sites were lower than scores for the parent-reported CBCL. This finding is consistent with findings from other studies (e.g., Herjanic, Herjanic, Brown, & Wheatt, 1975; Herjanic & Reich, 1982; Kazdin, Esveldt-Dawson, Unis, & Rancurello, 1983; Treiber & Mabe, 1987).

Children at both the Demonstration site and the Comparison site self-reported only slight (nonclinical) psychopathology on the YSR. Children at the Comparison site self-reported higher (worse) scores at Wave 1, although this difference between the sites was nonsignificant ($p = 0.11$). YSR

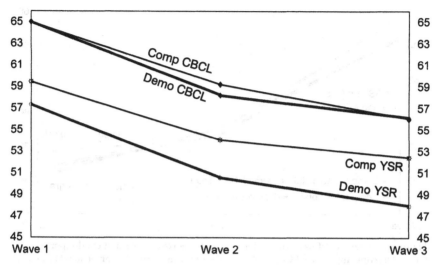

Figure 6.2. Measures of psychopathology: Parent-reported CBCL and child-reported YSR totals. All scores appear in CBCL-like standard scores with a Wave 1 mean of about 65 and SD = 10 for the whole sample. Nonclinic children have a mean of about 50 and SD = 10.

scores also dropped at both sites at Waves 2 and 3, but analysis of covariance revealed that on the basis of YSR scores alone, mental health outcome was significantly better at the Demonstration site. In Figure 6.2, superior YSR improvement in the Demonstration timeline can be seen in the steeper downward slope; with equal improvement over time, the Demonstration and Comparison timelines would be parallel. However, this observation was based on only one measure, and no conclusion should be drawn solely on the basis of a single test.

Figure 6.3 shows psychopathology outcome as measured by the Child Assessment Schedule (CAS) and the parent version (P-CAS). CAS and P-CAS psychopathology scores duplicated the overall pattern of improvement seen in Figure 6.2. However, statistically significant wave-by-site differences did not occur for the P-CAS or CAS as they did for the YSR.

Figures 6.4 and 6.5 display measures of functioning. These scores indicate social and behavioral functioning and are not related to psychiatric diagnosis. In Figure 6.4, CAS and P-CAS functioning totals (not related to psychiatric diagnosis) repeat the pattern of parallel improvement at both sites. There were no significant wave-by-site differences.

Figure 6.5 shows scores for the Child and Adolescent Functional Assessment Scale (CAFAS) and Global Level of Functioning (GLOF). Again, these measures of functioning repeated the pattern of improvement

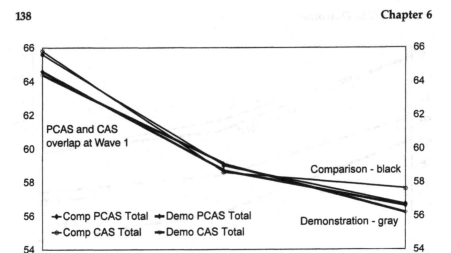

Figure 6.3. Measures of psychopathology: Parent-reported P-CAS and child-reported CAS totals. All scores appear in CBCL-like standard score with a Wave 1 mean of about 65 and SD = 10 for the whole sample. Nonclinic children have a mean of about 50 and SD = 10.

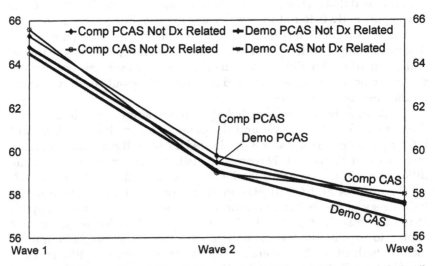

Figure 6.4. Measures of functioning: Parent-reported P-CAS and child-reported CAS. All scores appear in CBCL-like standard score with a Wave 1 mean of about 65 and SD = 10 for the whole sample. Nonclinic children have a mean of about 50 and SD = 10.

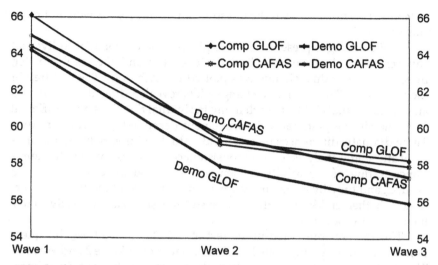

Figure 6.5. Functioning reported by parent and child: Interviewer-rated CAFAS and GLOF. All scores appear in CBCL-like standard score with a Wave 1 mean of about 65 and SD = 10 for the whole sample. Nonclinic children have a mean of about 50 and SD = 10.

seen on other measures. Scores at Wave 1 placed children at both sites in the clinical range, while at Waves 2 and 3, scores for children at both sites dropped into the nonclinical range. For the CAFAS, there were no wave-by-site differences. Children at the Demonstration site, however, exhibited better functioning at Wave 3 as measured by the GLOF; this difference was significant in the analysis of covariance.

Wave-by-site differences suggested that the average child improved and that there was a slight advantage for those treated in the Demonstration, as shown by significant differences on two of eight measures. A complete understanding of these clinical outcomes, however, required many more analyses before enough evidence was available to form a general conclusion.

INDIVIDUAL DIFFERENCES IN RESPONSE TO TREATMENT

Figures 6.2–6.5 show timelines on eight measures of mental health for 984 children in treatment. On all measures, the average child improved, but on only two of the eight were there significant site differences in outcome. This finding raises the question of why the results were not more consistent.

While averages present a simple picture, the outcome of individual children is much more complicated. To understand the results better, three-wave individual change was plotted for each of the 984 children in the Evaluation Sample. These change plots revealed dramatic differences among individual children, with many individual timelines quite different from the simple patterns of improvement described by sample means. These dramatic differences between individual children reduced the ability of any single analysis to draw consistent conclusions. Systematic significance testing of a carefully chosen list of key outcome measures was needed, and only by reviewing numerous results could the Project determine whether children at the Demonstration site had generally better mental health outcome.

The analyses presented in the rest of this chapter address this question: Did children at either site have better outcome at Wave 2 and Wave 3? The most powerful tests of these hypotheses were analyses of covariance. In addition to the analyses described below, a more advanced statistical approach to outcome analysis, the hierarchical linear modeling (HLM) of Bryk, Raudenbush, and Congdon (1994), was tested. This approach might be more powerful if the HLM model had fit the data precisely (S. W. Raudenbush, personal communication, July 1994).

Six total scores from the CAS and P-CAS were included in an HLM outcome analysis by Paul Greenbaum (personal communication, July 1994), a consultant experienced in its use. This HLM analysis found no significant site differences at Wave 2 or Wave 3. Therefore, the main outcome analyses were done with SAS General Linear Models using covariance analyses that corrected for pre-treatment differences at Wave 1.

DIAGNOSTIC CHANGE

Diagnostic Categories of the Child Assessment Schedule for Parents

One way to view outcomes is by the change in diagnosis between Waves 1 and 2 or between Waves 1 and 3. Presence or absence of diagnosis lacks the statistical power and precision of continuous measures, but this nominal view of outcome is direct, parsimonious, and reasonable. P-CAS diagnoses were chosen for analysis by the following criteria: frequency (diagnoses present in fewer than 10% of the sample at Wave 1 were not used), duplication (specific anxiety and depression categories were aggregated into "any depression" and "any anxiety"), and importance (adjustment reactions were not included in the analysis). These simplifications left six broad P-CAS diagnostic categories: attention-deficit disorder, conduct disorder, oppositional disorder, any anxiety, any depression, and enuresis. In addition, two higher-order P-CAS diagnostic categories were used: Any Diagnosis and Primary Diagnosis. All eight diagnostic categories were scored as "present" or "absent." This selection of P-CAS diagnoses was reviewed in terms of the seriousness of diagnosis by observing the correlation of each diagnosis with "severity," defined as the z-weighted sum of P-CAS psychopathology total and CAFAS functioning impairment. By this criterion, the adjustment diagnoses were the least serious (all having negative correlations with severity). The diagnoses of conduct disorder and "any depression" were the most serious diagnoses ($rs = 0.41$ and 0.31, respectively).

Outcome as Diagnostic Change

Therapeutic change in diagnosis was defined as "better" if the child received the diagnosis at Wave 1, but not on follow-up; "same" if the child had the diagnosis at Wave 1 and also on follow-up; or "worse" if the child lacked the diagnosis at Wave 1, but received it at follow-up.

Table 6.1 provides an example of diagnostic change for the conduct disorder diagnosis. Conduct disorder is one of the most serious diagnoses; it outranks all other P-CAS narrow-band diagnoses in its correlation with overall severity (P-CAS Total Psychopathology + CAFAS Functioning Impairment).

For children with the diagnosis of conduct disorder, there were nonsignificant differences in improvement between the Demonstration site and the Comparison site. There were more children with improved scores

Table 6.1. Diagnostic Outcome:
Conduct Disorder Diagnosis from Wave 1 to Wave 2
for 156 Children Having the Diagnosis

Site	Better (1,0)[a]	Same (1,1)[a]	Worse (0,1)[a]	Total
Demonstration	$N = 44$	$N = 27$	$N = 21$	$N = 92$
	47.8%	29.4%	22.8%	100%
Comparison	$N = 42$	$N = 12$	$N = 10$	$N = 64$
	65.6%	18.8%	15.6%	100%

[a]Better (1,0) means having the diagnosis on Wave 1 and lacking it on Wave 2; Same (1,1) means having the diagnosis at both waves; Worse (0,1) means lacking the diagnosis at Wave 1 and gaining it on Wave 2.

at the Comparison site (66%) than at the Demonstration site (48%), but this difference was not significant [$\chi^2(2) = 4.9$, $p = 0.09$]. This result was one of 16 statistical tests of the eight diagnostic measures at Waves 2 and 3. Table 6.2 summarizes 16 site-by-outcome (2×3) tables on the diagnostic outcome results for the six diagnoses and two summary diagnostic categories at Wave 2 and Wave 3.

Table 6.2 shows that there were no site differences in P-CAS diagnostic outcome, at either Wave 2 or Wave 3. This finding suggests no difference in outcome between the Demonstration and Comparison sites. Both sites had similar percentages of children who were "better" (having lost a diagnosis) or "worse" (having gained one). Most problems showed obvious improvement, with percentages of remission at Wave 3 above 50%. Indeed, even conduct disorder showed a 75% reduction at 1 year.

Figure 6.6 displays the time course of the two summary diagnostic categories for the Demonstration and Comparison sites and provides an overview of the mental health outcome for children in the Evaluation Sample. The top pair of timelines describes any diagnosis; nearly all children in treatment at both sites had some diagnosis at Wave 1. This percentage decreased over time, but at Wave 3, more than 80% of the children still had at least one diagnosis. Children improved at both sites, but few were free of mental health problems 1 year after intake.

The bottom pair of timelines in Figure 6.6 shows primary diagnosis, restricted to significant psychiatric disorders. At Wave 1, over 70% of children were seriously disturbed. The rate of serious psychopathology diminished to about 50% 1 year later, when about half the children were still seriously disturbed. In summary, 1 year after intake at both sites, over 80% of the children in the sample still had some diagnosable mental health problems, and half still had a serious mental health problem.

In conclusion, 16 analyses of diagnostic change suggested that the sites were about the same in their diagnostic rates of success.

PARENTS' OPINIONS ABOUT CHILDREN'S IMPROVEMENT

The children's primary caretakers (most often mothers) were asked to respond to five questions about their children's improvement at Wave 2 and Wave 3. A low score suggested that the child improved, while a high score suggested that the child became worse.

Both at Wave 2 and at Wave 3, these five items were quite consistent (Cronbach's $\alpha = 0.95$ at Wave 2, $\alpha = 0.94$ at Wave 3). Standardized αs and item αs were virtually identical, indicating that the items had such similar means and variances that item standardization was unnecessary. Outcome

Table 6.2. Change in P-CAS Diagnosis: Better or Worse by Site[a]

| Diagnosis | Wave 2 diagnostic change | | | | | Wave 3 diagnostic change | | | | | Probability | | | | Equality at Wave 1 | | |
| | N with Dx | Better | | Worse | | N with Dx | Better | | Worse | | $p(\chi^2)$ Wave 2 [χ^2 Wave 2] | $p(\chi^2)$ Wave 3 [χ^2 Wave 3] | | | Demo (N = 573) | Comp (N = 411) | $p(\chi^2)$ |
		Demo	Comp	Demo	Comp		Demo	Comp	Demo	Comp							
Attention-deficit	307	41%	41%	20%	18%	230	49%	42%	13%	18%	0.92	0.46			32%	31%	0.82
Conduct disorder	156	48%	66%	24%	16%	112	69%	79%	22%	15%	0.09	0.47			15%	17%	0.61
Oppositional	338	48%	45%	21%	24%	269	46%	43%	23%	26%	0.52	0.77			33%	32%	0.86
Anxiety, any	164	50%	61%	26%	27%	121	61%	69%	24%	20%	0.17	0.44			17%	12%	0.03[b]
Depression, any	276	57%	62%	24%	17%	216	65%	65%	18%	18%	0.41	0.96			27%	26%	0.77
Enuresis	98	30%	34%	15%	13%	77	45%	54%	14%	15%	0.66	0.68			11%	9%	0.24
Any diagnosis	771	9%	6%	1%	3%	608	12%	14%	1%	3%	0.10	0.18			98%	96%	0.14
Primary diagnosis	627	32%	35%	9%	6%	477	38%	39%	7%	3%	0.20	0.23			73%	72%	0.60

[a]To simplify the table, the category "percent unchanged" is not shown. Significance tests were done with χ^2 tests with 2 degrees of freedom on a 2×3 table, Site (Demonstration, Comparison) by Change (Better, Same, Worse). Ns in these analyses are fewer than 984 because (0,0) cases (those lacking the diagnosis at intake and at follow-up) were excluded. To make sure this limitation to outcome was not hiding site differences, the entire table was reanalyzed as a categorical repeated measures model with $N = 984$. The only significant result for this reanalysis was for "Any diagnosis" at Wave 2 ($p = 0.03$). Post-hoc reanalysis grouping "Any diagnosis" into "better" (1,0) vs. all others produced a near-significant result $\chi^2 = 3.64$, $p = 0.06$ favoring the Demonstration (7% "better" to 4% in the Comparison). The significant difference in equality at Wave 1 for "Any anxiety" shows that the rate of this diagnosis at the Demonstration site was significantly higher than at the Comparison site.
[b]Significant difference ($p < 0.05$).

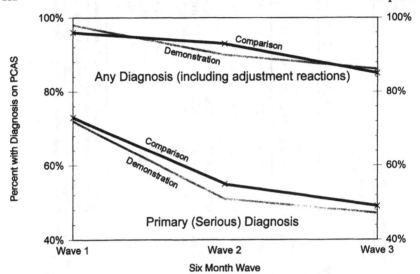

Figure 6.6. Percentages of the 984 children in the Evaluation Sample (573 at the Demonstration site and 411 at the Comparison site) with any diagnosis or a primary diagnosis at Wave 1.

was measured from two averages: the average of the five item scores at Wave 2 and the average of the five item scores at Wave 3. Table 6.3 presents descriptive statistics on these measures by site.

According to t-tests of the means, site differences were nonsignificant at Wave 2 ($p = 0.42$) and at Wave 3 ($p = 0.33$). There was no difference between sites in parents' opinions about their children's improvement during treatment. These results showing improvement but no site differences were consistent with those of standardized mental health measures, such as the CBCL and P-CAS.

Table 6.3. Parents' Rating
of Improvement by Site[a]

| | Mean improvement | | | |
| | Wave 2 ($N = 614$) | | Wave 3 ($N = 659$) | |
Site	Mean	SD	Mean	SD
Demonstration	9.22	4.36	9.44	4.20
Comparison	9.61	4.70	9.97	4.80

[a]A score of 10 would be an average of 2.0 ("a little better") per item. The Demonstration site's lower scores indicate better improvement than the Comparison site, but the standard deviations are so large that the differences may be due to change.

KEY MENTAL HEALTH MEASURES

In order to avoid undisciplined exploration of the many child and family variables in the data set, we chose a definitive list of outcome measures that should be influenced by superior mental health care. The 12 measures of mental health described in Table 6.4 represent this definitive list. The following brief discussion reviews these key outcome measures.

The most general single measure of a child's mental health status was "overall outcome," a composite score that combined child psychopathology, child functioning impairment, and family burden. This variable represented our assumption that effective mental health treatment should reduce child psychopathology (symptoms), increase a child's functioning competence, and reduce the emotional and logistical burden experienced by the families of troubled children. Thus, overall outcome was operationally defined as the z-weighted average of psychopathology as measured by the P-CAS, child functioning impairment as measured by the CAFAS, and parent-reported burden from the BCQ.

In addition to overall outcome, key mental health measures included seven total scores from core instruments and four individualized measures of the child's mental health. Individualized measures included the presenting problem as reported by both the parent and the child, and two measures of the most severe problem as reported by the parent and the child. The four individualized outcome variables were problem-focused, measuring only areas that were a particular problem for the child.

Table 6.5 presents descriptive statistics for the 12 key mental health outcome measures. The last two columns of Table 6.5 show the effect sizes of the change in means between Waves 1 and 2 and between Waves 2 and 3. The effect sizes for overall outcome of 0.65 and 0.31 show, for example, that the average child in the Evaluation Sample improved by 0.65 SD from Wave 1 to Wave 2, and improved a further 0.31 SD from Wave 2 to Wave 3.

Analysis of key outcome measures involved two phases. First, the 12 outcome measures were reduced to three simple categories (improved, same, worse) in an analysis very similar to that described above for diagnosis. Then more powerful analyses were conducted using continuous scores.

Reliable Change

Computing a Reliable Change Index (RCI) (Jacobson & Truax, 1991) offered a way to compare the Demonstration and Comparison sites in terms of how many children improved. For each of the 12 key outcome measures, each child's change score from Wave 1 to Wave 2, and also from Wave 1 to Wave 3, was classified as "improved," "unchanged," or

Table 6.4. Twelve Key Measures of Mental Health Outcome

Standardized measures	Description
Overall outcome (psychopathology + functioning + family burden)	z-weighted average of P-CAS psychopathology, CAFAS functioning impairment, and BCQ family burden. A single overall measure of outcome as reported by parent and scored by a trained rater. Psychopathology high.
Child Behavior Checklist (CBCL): Psychopathology total	Total psychopathology score from Achenbach's CBCL. Data reported directly by parent, scored with Achenbach's methods and norms. Widely used measure of child psychopathology. Psychopathology high.
Parent Child Assessment Schedule (P-CAS): Psychopathology total	Total psychopathology score from Hodges' P-CAS. Parent reports observations that are scored by a trained rater with ongoing reliability checks. Rigorous measure of child psychopathology in DSM-III-R terms. Psychopathology high.
Burden of Care (BCQ) total	Total burden (objective and subjective, internal and external) experienced by family as a result of having a troubled child. Measure of child's impact on the family that could be changed by effective treatment of the child. Psychopathology high.
Youth Self-Report (YSR): psychopathology total	Total psychopathology score from Achenbach's YSR, a variant of the CBCL self-reported by the child. Data reported directly by child, scored by Achenbach's methods and norms. Child-reported measures have fewer cases because only children 12 years old or older complete the YSR. Widely used measure of self-reported child psychopathology. Psychopathology high.
Child Assessment Schedule (CAS): Psychopathology total	Total psychopathology score from Hodges' CAS. Children report observations about themselves that are scored by a trained rater with ongoing reliability checks. Only children 8 years old or older take the CAS. Rigorous measure of child-reported psychopathology in DSM-III-R terms. Psychopathology high.
Child and Adolescent Functional Assessment Scale (CAFAS)	Overall functioning impairment from Hodges' CAFAS. Standardized rating of child functioning competence. Scored by a trained rater with ongoing reliability checks based on parent reports, child self-reports and all biographical data available to interviewer. Psychopathology high.
Global Level of Functioning (GLOF)	Global estimate of functioning at the month of interview. Scored by a trained rater with ongoing reliability checks based on parent reports, child self-reports, and all biographical data available to interviewer. Unlike other key variables, the GLOF is psychopathology low; a high score indicates functioning well.

(*continued*)

Table 6.4. (*Continued*)

Standardized measures	Description
Parent-reported individual measures	
Presenting problem: associated parent-reported psychopathology score	Using the parent's report of the child's main presenting problem, the corresponding parent-reported psychopathology score from the P-CAS is chosen to represent the child's key problem. Scores are standardized to eliminate differences among means of psychopathology measures.
Parent-reported "most severe" psychopathology	After psychopathology scores from the P-CAS and CBCL are standardized to the same mean and standard deviation, each child's highest (worst) score is chosen to represent his or her most severe mental health problem area.
Child-reported individualized measures	
Presenting problem: child-reported psychopathology score	Using the parent's report of the child's main presenting problem, the corresponding child-reported psychopathology score from the CAS is chosen to represent the child's key problem. Scores are standardized to eliminate differences among means of psychopathology measures.
Child-reported "most severe" psychopathology	After psychopathology scores from the CAS and YSR are standardized to the same mean and standard deviation, each child's highest (worst) score is chosen to represent his or her most severe self-reported mental health problem area.

"worse." Historically, change scores have been criticized (Cronbach & Furby, 1970), but recent methodological analysis (Newman, Reschovsky, Koneda, & Hendrick, 1994) recommends the difference score as a useful measure of change related to treatment.

Figure 6.7 shows the "improved," "same," and "worse" counts for overall outcome at Wave 3. At the Demonstration site, 84% of the children were improved at Wave 3; at the Comparison site, 88% were improved. An overall $\chi^2(2)$ for the two sites by three outcomes was nonsignificant [$p(\alpha)$ = 0.44 NS]. Thus, the counts of "improved," "same," and "worse" were about the same for the two sites. Two conclusions based on overall outcome scores at Wave 3 parallel results presented earlier; the majority of children improved and the percentage that improved was about the same at the Demonstration and Comparison sites.

An additional 23 analyses like the ones in Figure 6.7 compared rates of improvement at the Demonstration and Comparison sites on 12 key out-

Table 6.5. Descriptive Statistics for the 12 Key Outcome Measures

Outcome measure[a]	Wave 1 (intake)				Wave 2 (6 months)				Wave 3 (12 months)				Effect size[b]	
	Mean	SD	SEM	N	Mean	SD	SEM	N	Mean	SD	SEM	N	W1–W2	W2–W3
Overall outcome	65.01	10.01	0.33	932	58.56	9.89	0.37	730	55.61	9.09	0.38	567	0.65	0.31
CBCL psychopathology	65.17	10.38	0.34	924	58.55	11.85	0.42	804	56.05	12.21	0.46	694	0.60	0.21
P-CAS psychopathology total	29.82	13.91	0.44	984	21.43	13.56	0.49	781	18.68	12.71	0.51	617	0.61	0.21
BCQ total	2.48	0.82	0.03	932	2.17	0.81	0.03	770	1.94	0.74	0.03	656	0.38	0.30
YSR psychopathology total	58.61	10.87	0.54	412	52.33	11.37	0.59	375	50.54	11.93	0.65	341	0.56	0.15
CAS psychopathology total	22.21	12.95	0.50	675	15.10	10.99	0.47	557	12.18	10.24	0.47	471	0.59	0.28
CAFAS functioning competence	45.65	26.47	0.84	984	31.40	26.03	0.93	781	25.51	23.83	0.96	617	0.54	0.24
GLOF	3.29	0.86	0.03	980	3.85	0.93	0.03	777	4.00	0.92	0.04	613	−0.63	−0.16
Presenting problem: Parent-reported	66.72	8.47	0.27	970	65.25	7.92	0.29	769	60.89	7.06	0.29	607	0.55	0.18
Parent-reported "most severe" psychopathology[c]	80.24	9.39	0.30	984	68.07	11.23	0.40	790	65.42	10.46	0.41	655	1.18[c]	0.24
Presenting problem: Child-reported	63.65	8.94	0.35	665	59.67	6.92	0.30	547	58.29	6.23	0.29	463	0.50	0.21
Child-reported "most severe" psychopathology[c]	77.26	11.03	0.42	684	64.49	10.25	0.45	508	62.38	9.57	0.47	414	1.20[c]	0.21

[a]Higher GLOF scores indicate less impairment; for all other scales, higher scores indicate more impairment.
[b]Effect size measured in SDs.
[c]The inflated W1–W2 effect sizes for "most severe" psychopathology may be due to regression. Choosing the highest scores may increase the W1–W2 effect sizes for purely statistical reasons.

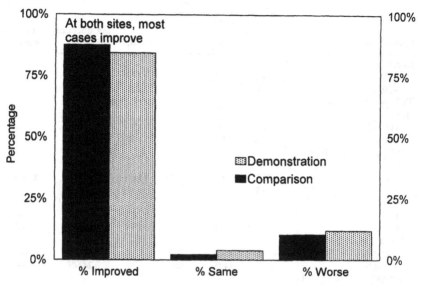

Figure 6.7. Overall outcome: Clinical improvement in children at the Demonstration and Comparison sites at Wave 3.

come measures at Waves 2 and 3. Results of all 24 analyses are presented in Table 6.6.

Only 3 of the 24 analyses of improvement showed any significant differences between the Demonstration and Comparison sites. One would expect about 1 of 20 tests to be statistically significant by chance alone. These significant differences all favored the Comparison site. Since these differences occurred at Wave 2 but not at Wave 3, the Comparison site children improved faster, but were not better at 1 year on these three measures. Overall, then, these results showed that:

- Most children improved at Waves 2 and 3.
- Improvement rates were somewhat higher by Wave 3 than by Wave 2.
- There were few significant site differences (3 of 24), only slightly more than chance (1 of 20).
- The three significant site differences favored the Comparison site at Wave 2.

The results suggest that mental health outcome was about equal at the two sites.

Table 6.6. Reliable Change at the Demonstration and Comparison Sites

	Outcome[a]					
	Improved		Worse		Significance	Better
Outcome measure[b]	Demo	Comp	Demo	Comp	$\chi^2(2)$	outcome
Overall outcome						
Wave 2	76%	78%	20%	18%	0.70NS	—
Wave 3	84%	88%	12%	10%	0.44NS	—
CBCL psychopathology total						
Wave 2	74%	76%	21%	20%	0.92NS	—
Wave 3	82%	81%	16%	15%	0.86NS	—
P-CAS psychopathology total						
Wave 2	73%	78%	25%	18%	0.04[c]	Comp
Wave 3	80%	81%	15%	13%	0.78NS	—
BCQ total						
Wave 2	63%	68%	27%	24%	0.29NS	—
Wave 3	73%	80%	19%	15%	0.07NS	—
YSR total psychopathology						
Wave 2	70%	64%	20%	22%	0.42NS	—
Wave 3	74%	68%	15%	2%	0.24NS	—
CAS psychopathology total						
Wave 2	66%	76%	23%	15%	0.03[c]	Comp
Wave 3	78%	81%	13%	13%	0.39NS	—
CAFAS functioning						
Wave 2	62%	64%	23%	23%	0.79NS	—
Wave 3	73%	70%	16%	17%	0.65NS	—
GLOF						
Wave 2	49%	49%	14%	13%	0.77NS	—
Wave 3	55%	54%	13%	10%	0.43NS	—
Presenting problem: parent-reported						
Wave 2	67%	73%	24%	18%	0.13NS	—
Wave 3	74%	79%	19%	14%	0.20NS	—
Parent-reported "most severe" psychopathology						
Wave 2	82%	85%	7%	6%	0.35NS	—
Wave 3	88%	90%	5%	4%	0.56NS	—
Presenting problem: Child-reported						
Wave 2	60%	72%	25%	22%	0.005[d]	Comp
Wave 3	71%	72%	19%	19%	0.98NS	—
Child-reported "most severe" psychopathology						
Wave 2	80%	85%	6%	6%	0.24NS	—
Wave 3	87%	88%	6%	5%	0.96NS	—

[a]The percentage unchanged is not shown: improved (RCI more than +2) + unchanged (RCI −2 to +2) + worse (RCI less than −2) = 100%. RCI = change score/SE of change score.
[b]All scales are pathology high except the GLOF.
[c]$p < 0.05$.
[d]$p < 0.01$.

CONTINUOUS MEASURES OF OUTCOME

Outcome at Wave 2

The failure to find site differences in two categorical analyses (diagnosis and reliable change) was not in itself convincing evidence that there were no site differences in outcome, since categorical measures of outcome are less precise than exact measurements (Maxwell & Delaney, 1993). For example, the P-CAS Major Depression symptom count is more informative than the sheer presence or absence of that diagnosis. Table 6.7 presents site differences in outcome on continuous measures at Wave 2.

Overall site superiority results appear in the rightmost column of Table 6.7. In this table, analysis of YSR psychopathology favored the Demonstration site. Two other outcomes were significant, both favoring the Comparison site; on the child-reported CAS psychopathology total and the child-reported psychopathology scale that fit the child's presenting problem, children improved more at the Comparison site than they did at the Demonstration site. However, it is possible that the site difference favoring the Comparison site was a by-product of the Comparison site's exhibiting significantly more pathological scores at Wave 1. Analysis of covariance minimizes such differences statistically, but the most prudent interpretation of the CAS site effect is as a "probable result favoring the Comparison site." The child-reported presenting problem result was not confounded by Wave 1 differences, but its significance was modest ($p = 0.04$). Both differences favoring the Comparison site were small (ES = 0.19 SD). Overall, given the preponderance of nonsignificant differences, and the small effect sizes, the results at Wave 2 appear very close to equal for the two sites.

Summary of Mental Health Outcomes at Wave 2

In summary, several significant differences between the Demonstration and Comparison sites appeared at Wave 2:

- Among 12 key outcome measures there were 3 significant differences.
- Two differences favored the Comparison site, one the Demonstration site.
- According to the child-reported YSR total psychopathology, children 12 years old and older improved more at the Demonstration site.
- According to the child-reported CAS total, children 8 years old and older improved more at the Comparison site.

Table 6.7. Statistical Summary: Overall Outcome Site Effects at Wave 2

Outcome measure[a]	Statistical problems		Outcome at Wave 2						
	Wave 1 interactions $p(\alpha)$	Wave 1 differences $p(\alpha)$	Demonstration site		Comparison site		$Prob(\alpha)$	Effect sizes of significant differences	Superior outcome site
			Mean	SEM	Mean	SEM			
Overall outcome	NS	0.95	58.9	0.36	58.3	0.42	0.22		Neither
CBCL psychopathology total	NS	0.82	57.9	0.44	59.2	0.48	0.51		Neither
P-CAS psychopathology total	NS	0.13	21.7	0.49	21.0	0.57	0.35		Neither
BCQ total	NS	0.62	2.2	0.03	2.2	0.04	0.35		Neither
YSR psychopathology total	NS	0.11	51.2	0.71	53.4	0.75	0.03[c]	0.25 SD	Demo
CAS psychopathology total	NS	0.02[b]	15.3	0.52	13.5	0.62	0.03[c]	0.19 SD	Comp
CAFAS functioning competence	NS	0.08	31.8	1.10	30.8	1.3	0.52		Neither
GLOF	NS	0.03	3.9	0.04	3.8	0.05	0.30		Neither
Presenting problem: parent-reported	NS	0.12	62.4	0.31	61.9	0.36	0.27		Neither
Parent-reported "most severe" psychopathology	NS	0.37	68.1	0.47	68.0	0.54	0.80		Neither
Presenting problem: child-reported	NS	0.13	60.0	0.34	58.9	0.40	0.04[c]	0.19 SD	Comp
Child-reported "most severe" psychopathology	NS	0.19	64.3	0.52	64.8	0.61	0.57		Neither

[a] All scores are pathology high except the GLOF.
[b] The Demonstration site is lower at Wave 1.
[c] Significant difference.

- According to child-reported CAS presenting-problem psychopathology, children 8 years old and older improved more at the Comparison site.

Outcome at Wave 3

As shown in Table 6.8, there were 2 significant site differences in outcome at Wave 3. Children at the Demonstration site had better outcome on both the YSR and the GLOF. For the YSR, the Demonstration site had a 0.35 SD superiority in outcome. For the GLOF, the Demonstration site had a 0.21 SD superiority over the Comparison site. According to Lipsey (1990), both of these effect sizes are small for evaluative research. However, this finding of 2 of 12 results favoring the Demonstration site is more than one would expect by chance.

Summary of Mental Health Outcomes at Wave 3

At Wave 3, the following site differences were found:

- There was significantly better outcome favoring the Demonstration site for YSR total score. The difference between corrected means was small (effect size = 0.35 SD).
- There was significantly better outcome at the Demonstration site on the GLOF for children of all ages. The difference between corrected means was small (effect size = 0.21 SD).

SUMMARY OF OVERALL MENTAL HEALTH OUTCOME

Program theory predicted better outcome in the Demonstration site at both Wave 2 and Wave 3 (quicker recovery, better outcome). At Wave 2, there were three small site differences, with two favoring the Comparison site. At Wave 3, there were two results, both favoring the Demonstration site. At both Waves 2 and 3, the YSR total score favored the Demonstration site, so it may be considered a repeated result. In addition, at Wave 3, the GLOF favored the Demonstration site.

These results reveal a slight statistical advantage of the Demonstration site in three ways:

- A box score count favored the Demonstration site 3–2.
- YSR results favoring the Demonstration site were found at both Waves 2 and 3.
- The two results favoring the Comparison site involved very small effect sizes.

Table 6.8. Statistical Summary: Overall Outcome Site Effects at Wave 3

Outcome measure[a]	Statistical problems		Outcome at Wave 2					Effect sizes of significant differences	Superior outcome site
	Wave 1 interactions p(α)	Wave 1 differences p(α)	Demonstration site		Comparison site		Prob(α)		
			Mean	SEM	Mean	SEM			
Overall outcome	NS	0.31	55.7	0.42	55.8	0.49	0.87		Neither
CBCL psychopathology total	NS	0.78	55.6	0.51	56.3	0.55	0.33		Neither
P-CAS psychopathology total	NS	0.14	18.5	0.56	18.9	0.65	0.68		Neither
BCQ total	NS	0.08	1.9	0.04	1.9	0.03	0.35		Neither
YSR psychopathology total	NS	0.25	48.3	0.97	52.1	0.92	0.01[b]	0.35 SD	Demo
CAS psychopathology total	NS	0.02[b]	11.6	0.56	11.5	0.62	0.84		Neither
CAFAS functioning competence	NS	0.68	24.1	1.20	27.4	1.4	0.07		Neither
GLOF	0.03	0.02	4.1	0.05	4.0	0.06	0.03[b]	0.21 SD	Demo
Presenting problem: parent-reported	NS	0.11	60.9	0.33	60.9	0.38	0.99		Neither
Parent-reported "most severe" psychopathology	NS	0.67	65.7	0.49	65.1	0.56	0.40		Neither
Presenting problem: child-reported	NS	0.34	58.1	0.37	58.0	0.42	0.71		Neither
Child-reported "most severe" psychopathology	NS	0.15	62.1	0.59	62.8	0.66	0.42		Neither

[a]All scores are pathology high except the GLOF.
[b]Significant difference.

On a practical level, however, finding 5 small bidirectional differences among 24 tests suggests that outcome is very close to equal at the Demonstration and Comparison sites.

The significance of these findings may be examined from three viewpoints: statistical significance, clinical significance, and significance for mental health policy. Statistically, there were a handful of significant differences, a few more than one would expect by chance. The paucity of repeated significant results was not satisfying, and there were only a few more differences than one finds in random numbers. Clinical significance is more important: Did the observed results suggest site differences that a clinician could detect? The results are clinically disappointing, since the observed differences were very small and did not replicate across respondents. The YSR results, for example, had an effect size of 0.25 SD at Wave 2 and 0.35 SD at Wave 3. An example of difference of 0.30 SD would be a t-score of 53 vs. 50, a small difference. A few scattered results, mainly in child self-reports that did not replicate across instruments (the YSR and CAS), or, more important, results that did not converge across respondents, cannot be considered clinically significant. It is unlikely that an expert clinician reviewing these results would advise, "Send the child to the Demonstration site. The results are better there by 0.30 SD on two of the twelve measures."

The third and most stringent level of significance is at the level of policy. So far, there is no pattern of results so one-sided that one would conclude that either site offers a system of care with superior clinical outcomes that serve as a model for national policy. Policymakers judging possible systems of mental health care for children and adolescents cannot look to these small differences in outcome to decide whether the Demonstration site or the Comparison site offers better results for children. The outcomes are virtually identical from a policy point of view.

CONCLUSIONS: OVERALL OUTCOME

In sum, these conclusions can be drawn:

- Children at both sites improved.
- There was no superiority in mental health outcome at the Demonstration site. Whatever its other virtues, the continuum of care did not result in better scores on mental health outcome measures.
- Outcome was studied in a variety of ways. While results showed slightly more site differences than would be expected by chance, those differences favored the Comparison site about as often as the Demonstration site.

The results presented above addressed the general Demonstration hypothesis that children in the Demonstration site, as a whole, would improve more than children treated at the Comparison site. The following section studies particular subgroups of children to see whether there are subgroups for whom the hypothesis of superior outcome at the Demonstration site holds. In particular, ten specific hypotheses were developed that predicted that certain children would have better clinical outcomes in the Demonstration site. These hypotheses are presented and explained in Table 6.9.

Five Theory-Driven Hypotheses

The sections that follow repeat the analysis of the 12 key outcome measures using the same analytical paradigm. Each analysis follows the question it was conducted to answer.

Intermediate Care

Will children who need intermediate care (more-than-outpatient office sessions but less than hospital treatment) have better outcomes in the Demonstration?

Operationally, one of the most dramatic differences between Demonstration and Comparison sites is the provision of intermediate levels of care. If the Demonstration site achieved better outcomes, it should have done so with children who needed these intermediate levels of care. To test this hypothesis, children in the entire Evaluation Sample were divided into two groups, based on whether they needed intermediate care or not. Children who needed intermediate care were identified by their clinical characteristics. First, the clinical characteristics of Demonstration children actually receiving such care were determined by logistic regression. Next, a score was calculated for every child in both sites indicating how closely he or she resembled the intermediate clinical profile. Finally, cases were assigned to "intermediate" or "not intermediate" groups on the basis of a cutting score that minimized site differences in sensitivity–specificity analysis. The accuracy of this procedure was less than 50% among Demonstration children receiving such care, and about 80% accurate among those not receiving intermediate care.

Among the four significant results of the intermediate outcome analysis, two favored the Demonstration site, two the Comparison site. Two subgroups of Comparison children were seen by their caretakers as improving more by Wave 2 than similar groups of Demonstration children. Two subgroups of Demonstration children improved more than Comparison youth by Wave 3. These mixed differences among 24 outcome analyses suggested a very slight advantage of the Demonstration site, where the two significant superior outcomes occurred at Wave 3. The overall conclusion from this analysis, however, was equal mental health outcomes at the Demonstration and Comparison sites.

More-Than-Outpatient Treatment

Will children who need more-than-outpatient treatment (either intermediate or hospital care) have better outcomes in the Demonstration?

This outcome analysis defined need for more-than-outpatient treatment. Logistic regression established the best clinical predictors for more-than-outpatient treatment. This equation was then used to classify all children at both the Demonstration and Comparison sites as needing or not-needing more-than-outpatient care.

There were no significant site differences on any of the 12 key outcome measures at either Wave 2 or Wave 3.

Severity

Will the most severe[1] cases, those with high psychopathology combined with high functioning impairment, have better outcome in the Demonstration?

The severity hypothesis concerns children's overall mental health status on intake, as defined by the z-weighted average of psychopathology (P-CAS) and functioning impairment (CAFAS). There were no site differences in an analysis of outcome by severity of overall psychopathology.

Pervasive Child Psychopathology

Will children whose psychopathology is pervasive (symptomatic of many diagnoses) have better outcomes in the Demonstration?

"Pervasiveness" was defined as the number of narrow-band scales that were clinically elevated for a child. For example, for parent-reported psychopathology (CBCL and P-CAS), pervasiveness was a count of the number of scales that were clinically elevated. Three measures of pervasiveness (parent-reported, child-reported, and interviewer-rated) were

---

[1]Another approach to severity would be to add quadratic or cubic terms to the overall outcome model. Squaring or cubing the Wave 1 covariate would add nonlinear terms that emphasized outliers. These analyses produced some of the same results, and no new site effects, when compared with the overall analyses of 12 key outcome measures at Wave 3.

Table 6.9. Hypotheses for Site Differences in Outcome

Class of hypothesis	Clinical group	Hypothesis	Rationale
General demonstration hypothesis	All children ages 5–17	Children who enter treatment at the Demonstration site will have better clinical improvement at 6 and 12 months than children at the Comparison site	The Demonstration site's continuum of care offers a range of services appropriate for cases from mild to severe. Traditional care offers no intermediate services, haphazard assignment of cases, and no mechnism for continuity of care with multiple services.
Theory-driven subgroup analysis	Children who need intermediate services (with or without hospitalization)	Such children will show greater improvement, or improve more quickly, at the Demonstration site.	No intermediate services are offered at the Comparison site, so children who need them received less appropriate outpatient or inpatient care.
	Children with severe mental health problems	Such children will show greater improvement, or improve more quickly, at the Demonstration site.	The Demonstration site's full range of services will benefit children who need multiple services and smooth transitions between them. Children with milder mental health problems who need only a few outpatient sessions may get equal care in the Demonstration and Comparison sites.
	Children with pervasive multidiagnosis problems	Such children will show greater improvement, or improve more quickly, at the Demonstration site.	Children with multiple problems are more likely to need a complex combination of services, including intermediate services not available in traditional mental health care.

Children with multiple problems	Such children will show greater improvement, or improve more quickly, at the Demonstration site.	Children from such families are more likely to need a mix of services. Each service must be sought out individually by families in traditional care, but these families are less able to do so. A continuum of care provides the service coordination needed by these families.
Basic exploratory hypotheses Children vs. teens	Demonstration and Comparison site outcomes may differ for children vs. teens.	Children (5–12) and teens (13–18) have distinct age-related problems, different relationships with their parents, and different treatment needs. Thus, teens and children may not respond in the same way to the two different treatment programs.
Males vs. females	Demonstration and Comparison site outcomes may differ for males vs. females.	Male and female children, to some extent, have different mental health problems and different treatment needs (e.g., attention-deficit disorder and conduct problems in males, depression and anorexia in females). Thus, to the extent that treatment programs inadvertently favor a gender, males and females might not respond in the same way to services at the Demonstration and Comparison sites.

averaged into an overall index. A child with a high score on general pervasiveness had problems in the range of clinical severity affecting a number of separate functioning areas. Out of 24 outcome analyses, there was 1 significant result: Comparison-site children with more pervasive impairment reported greater improvement in the presenting-problem area than Demonstration-site children. Otherwise, pervasiveness of psychopathology had no influence on site differences in outcome. Finding 1 site difference among 24 analyses may be interpreted as approximately equal results.

Children with Multiple Problems

Will children with multiple problems—complex cases including pervasive child psychopathology, family stress, and reduced family resources—have better outcomes in the Demonstration?

If a child with serious problems who needs a mix of services comes from a family with other problems, the Demonstration has many more ways in which to respond.

The "multiproblem" construct was defined as broadly as possible to include both multiply troubled children and multiply stressed parents. It included:

- Breadth of the child's problems—the z-weighted average of the number of systems in which the child was treated (mental health, education, or juvenile justice), the number of settings in which the child had difficulties, and the pervasiveness of the child's symptoms, as seen by parent, child, and interviewer.
- Poor family resources—the z-weighted average of Family Resource Scale and Family Index of Regenerativity and Adaptation family resource problems.
- High family stress—the z-weighted average of Family Assessment Device and Family Inventory of Life Events totals.

A multidimensional index was defined as the z-weighted average of scores for pervasiveness, poor family resources, and stress. Before use, the multiproblem total was standardized to a mean of 65, with an SD of 10, at Wave 1. Standardized scores were converted into the "psychopathology-high" direction when necessary. A "multiple-problem case" was defined as one in the top 25% of the total sample on the multiple problem sum.

There were no significant Wave 2 or Wave 3 site differences resulting from the number of multiple mental health problems at intake.

Conclusion: Five Theory-Driven Hypotheses

Five outcome analyses were conducted, searching for site differences predicted from program theory. Superior outcome at the Demonstration site was predicted for the groups of children who needed intermediate care but not hospital care, children who needed more treatment than outpatient sessions, children with severe psychopathology and impairment, children from families with multiple problems, and children with pervasive psychopathology (as opposed to single-problem children).

In each analysis, outcome was measured by 12 key outcome measures at Wave 2 and Wave 3. While there were slightly more findings than expected from chance alone, observed differences equally favored the Demonstration and Comparison sites.

Basic Exploratory Hypotheses

In addition to the theory-driven hypotheses, subgroups based on age and gender were studied.

Children vs. Teens

When the 12 key outcome measures were tested for age-by-site interactions, there were no age-related site differences at Wave 2. At Wave 3, of four significant site differences by age, two favored the Comparison site and two favored the Demonstration site. These few differences do not support the overall superiority of either site for younger or older clients.

Males vs. Females

When the 12 key outcome measures were tested for site interactions, only one significant site interaction occurred. Contrasts of site effects within this interaction suggested that males' most severe problems were improved slightly more at Wave 3 at the Demonstration site. There were no significant site differences for females. Finding 1 difference among 24 tests suggests that the sites are about equal in outcome.

OVERALL CONCLUSIONS

When mental health outcome was analyzed from a variety of points of view, the following results were found:

- The average child improved at either site;
- The amount of mental health improvement was about the same at either site;
- Subgroups of children hypothesized to have better outcome in the Demonstration enjoyed the same amount of improvement at the Comparison site.

The Outcome Study did not find support for the hypothesis that the Demonstration's system of care led to better mental health outcome than the traditional system of services at the Comparison site.

7

Cost Outcomes

This chapter examines one of the ultimate outcomes of the program model: costs (see Figure 7.1). It considers whether care provided under the continuum of care is less expensive than under traditional systems. It presents Demonstration cost data and offers and explains between-site cost comparisons. This discussion focuses on seven questions:

1. As a system of care, was the Demonstration more costly?
2. Did the distribution of expenditures across children and services differ between sites?
3. What explains the difference in system-level costs?
4. Why do average expenditures per treated child differ?
5. Were intermediate services substituted for more expensive and restrictive services?
6. Are the differences in average expenditures per treated child due to differences in the mix of children treated?
7. How did the Demonstration affect costs outside the specialty mental health sector?

Before considering these questions, however, we provide a conceptual overview of the costs of children's mental illness. This overview provides a context in which to place our findings. A summary and discussion concludes the chapter.

DEFINITION OF COSTS

Economics generally measures the costs of an activity by the effect it has on the total resources available for alternative uses. This broad defini-

163

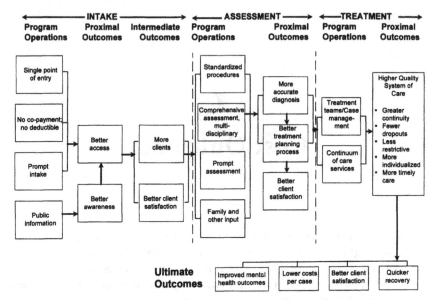

Figure 7.1. Fort Bragg Child and Adolescent Demonstration: Program theory.

tion of costs recognizes that the effects of a program or illness may have a variety of effects. Economists generally group the resulting costs into two categories: direct costs and indirect costs. Direct costs "are closely related to the primary objectives of the project"; indirect costs are "byproducts, multipliers, [or] spillovers" of the project (Kee, 1994, p. 466). Direct costs tend to involve resources purchased to run the program, while indirect costs involve resources consumed incidentally (Warner & Luce, 1982, p. 77).

This distinction is especially useful in a discussion of mental illness or of the effects of mental health services (McGuire, 1991; Rice et al., 1990; Wyatt & Clark, 1987). Direct costs of mental health care are the visible expenses of treatment (e.g., the costs of an hour of psychotherapy). These costs may be incurred both within and outside the specialty mental health sector. Examples of the latter include care received from a medical practitioner or a school counselor.

Indirect mental health costs involve value of "lost output due to the reduced or lost productivity caused by illness, disability, or injury" (McGuire, 1991, p. 375). These costs include, for example, the time parents miss from work because they are caring for the child. Other indirect costs also include damage the child does to physical property or to himself or herself or to another person.

This overview of the costs of mental disorders provides a context in which to place the results of the Project's Cost Study. It highlights the fact that Project analyses focused on an important but limited subset of total costs: direct costs incurred in the specialty mental health sector. The data on other costs—indirect costs and direct costs incurred elsewhere—are very limited. Two such costs seem especially important: the costs of treatment that children received in the juvenile justice and other systems and the costs of not treating children.

Ignoring these costs provides a somewhat limited view of the costs of the continuum of care. Such a system may lower the costs of mental illness by increasing direct expenditures on mental health services but lowering costs elsewhere. Focusing only on direct expenditures on specialty mental health services may lead one to conclude incorrectly that a socially beneficial policy increases the costs of mental illness.

It is important to note that, for some purposes, focusing on expenditures on mental health services is appropriate. If one's perspective is that of the agency (e.g., the Army) or the persons (e.g., parents) financing the services, such a focus is indeed correct. It is largely irrelevant that higher expenditures on mental health services may have been offset elsewhere. The burden on that particular agency or person has increased.

Is there any reason to believe that the costs of mental illness outside the specialty mental health sector differed between sites? Evidence indicates that some children eligible for the Civilian Health and Medical Program of the Uniformed Services (CHAMPUS) at Fort Campbell were hospitalized in State facilities in Tennessee with the encouragement of the military treatment facility (see Chapter 2). If so, CHAMPUS costs understate the total costs of treating children at the Comparison site. The Demonstration's "no reject, no eject" philosophy may have meant that those children would have been treated within the system under the Demonstration. In that case, the costs at the Comparison site are lower not because caring for those children was less costly for society but because the Army shifted costs to the State of Tennessee. Similarly, the provision of therapeutic foster and group homes may have reduced public expenditures on foster care.

While these costs lie outside the main sources of data for the Cost Study [CHAMPUS and the Demonstration Management Information System (MIS)], supplemental data were collected to gauge their magnitude. As noted in Chapter 2, the State of Tennessee provided the Project with information on CHAMPUS-eligible children treated in State facilities. In addition, information was available from the Evaluation Sample about damage caused to property and injuries inflicted on self and others. Information was also available from parents on services children received in other settings (e.g., contact with law enforcement). The last question considered focuses on these costs and on how they affect the overall costliness of the Demonstration.

This brief discussion of costs highlights a second feature of the Cost Study: The figures presented here are best labeled "expenditures." The key distinction between the two involves the treatment of excess profits producers earn (as used here, "excess" profits refer to "economic" profits or profits above and beyond the economy-wide average rate of profit). Economists define the costs of an activity in terms of its claim on society's resources; to the extent that the activity transfers those resources from one member of society to another, no costs are incurred. Excess profits represent such a transfer; while these payments impose a burden on the consumers involved, they do not reduce the pool of resources society has available for other uses.

Basic economics suggests that these profits can be substantial in a noncompetitive market such as the one for mental health services (Folland, Goodman, & Stano, 1993). Because these profits do not represent resources used (they are transfers from one group of society to another), they should be excluded from cost calculations (Gramlich, 1981).

This distinction has two implications. For both sites, expenditures on mental health services are likely to exceed the costs to society of providing those services to children and adolescents. A second implication, however, is potentially more important. If the gap between costs and expenditures differs between sites, the relative costliness of the Demonstration is misstated. In particular, if the gap between costs and expenditures is smaller at the Demonstration site, the expenditure figures presented here understate the extent to which costs at the Demonstration site exceed those at the Comparison site. (Producing cost figures for both sites would require one to subtract greater excess profits from expenditures at the Comparison site. This adjustment would increase the gap between sites still further.)

There is some evidence that this gap is understated. Cardinal negotiated rates for externally provided services that were 90% of the corresponding CHAMPUS charges. It is possible that by offering increased volumes of services, Cardinal was able to negotiate charges closer to the underlying costs of producing the services. In addition, for internally provided services, expenditure figures here represent the actual costs of services.

Thus, the figures presented here likely overstate the social costs of providing children with mental health services. It also seems likely that the differences in expenditures presented here understate actual between-site differences in costs per se; i.e., the differences in direct costs between sites are probably larger than the differences in expenditures on mental health services reported later in this chapter.

QUESTION 1. AS A SYSTEM OF CARE, WAS THE DEMONSTRATION MORE COSTLY?

This section considers overall expenditures at the Demonstration and Comparison sites. It also examines the services on which and the children in whose behalf expenditures were made and the adjustments in total expenditures that one might make to more fully account for between-site differences.

Table 7.1 presents total expenditures for fiscal years 1988–1993 as well as for the Demonstration period (fiscal years 1991–1993) as a whole. Expenditures on mental health services under the Demonstration were dramatically higher than those under traditional services. This difference hold true whether we compare those expenditures to those prior to the Demonstration in the Fort Bragg catchment area or to those at the Comparison site for the same period of time.

During the course of the Demonstration, expenditures on mental health services tallied $50 million. Expenditures during the Demonstration period totaled $47 million, and an additional $2 million was spent during the startup period (the last half of fiscal year 1990). This amount is triple the

Table 7.1. Total and Average Costs per Treated Child and Costs per Eligible Child[a]

	Demonstration site			Comparison site		
Period	Total costs	Costs/ client	Costs/ eligible	Total costs	Costs/ client	Costs/ eligible
Fiscal year						
1988	$3,842,087	$4,096	$100	$7,942,651	$8,369	$200
1989	4,558,480	4,056	111	8,486,255	7,137	195
1990 (CHAMPUS)	3,708,337	3,329	87	8,483,363	6,830	199
1990	2,033,804	2,631	48	Transition period		
1991	13,307,209	5,025	299	6,954,818	$5,261	$152
1992	16,245,926	4,883	353	3,193,966	2,883	85
1993	17,365,676	4,862	387	3,474,492	3,034	79
Demonstration period	46,918,811	7,777	1,056	13,633,749	4,904	321

[a]These data describe the treated population at the Demonstration and Comparison sites. The Demonstration period is the combined fiscal years 1991–1993.

amount spent at the Comparison site during the same period.[1] Expenditures in fiscal year 1993 (over $17 million) were 4.5 times those for fiscal year 1989, the year prior to Demonstration start-up.

Perhaps more striking, however, are expenditures per eligible child. On average, children eligible for care at the Demonstration received over $1000 in services. This is 3 times the amount for children treated at the Comparison site.

As discussed earlier, parents bore none of the costs of care at the Demonstration site, but did pay roughly 10% of the total costs at the Comparison site. Therefore, aggregate expenditures hide the fact that Army costs at the Comparison site are actually lower than total expenditures. In particular, Army costs are 90% of the figures reported in Table 7.1. Total Army costs were $12,381,346; average Army costs per client, $4545. From the Army's perspective, therefore, the effect of the Demonstration on costs is even greater than that reported in Table 7.1. The analyses that follow focus on total expenditures, regardless of whether the Army or parents were the source of payment. The distribution of expenditures between parents and the Army is a separate issue: It involves a transfer of income from parents to the Army. The key question is whether the continuum of care is more or less costly for society. The issue of who should bear those costs is distinct and not considered here.

The expenditure figures cited here seem enormous. Another way of expressing them is as costs per eligible child. Table 7.1 shows that by the end of the Demonstration period, average yearly expenditures per eligible child were nearly $400 at the Demonstration site. Thus, an average of $400 had to be set aside for each of the children in the catchment area, whether they received mental health services or not. This figure is nearly 5 times that for the Comparison site. This discrepancy is especially striking given that prior to the Demonstration, average expenditures per eligible child were higher at the Comparison site.

We considered four potential adjustments to our data. These adjustments reflect differences between sites not accounted for in simple comparisons of CHAMPUS with Rumbaugh Clinic MIS data. These adjustments involve (1) the administrative costs of managing the CHAMPUS system, (2) expenditures by CHAMPUS on services provided during the

---

[1] A case could be made that the costs of services at the Comparison site should be calculated using the per-unit CHAMPUS charges for the Fort Bragg catchment area. Using charges from the Comparison site confounds cost differences due to differences in service utilization with those due to differences in per-unit costs that may have existed even in the absence of the Demonstration. This point, however, has no practical implications; using the per-unit costs from the Fort Bragg catchment area raises total costs (and cost per treated child) at the Comparison site by less than 0.25%.

Demonstration period to children in the Fort Bragg catchment area, (3) the costs of services delivered under the Gateway to Care system, and (4) the treatment of costs associated with the Demonstration's status as a Demonstration Project. We consider each of these in turn. Table 7.2 demonstrates the effect of each on the overall cost picture.

The figures in Table 7.1 include the costs of managing Rumbaugh Clinic but ignore the costs of administering the CHAMPUS system. These costs principally involved the costs of processing claims and of performing the precertification and continuing care reviews. The task of processing claims was performed by a fiscal intermediary (FI) that charged between $6.08 and $6.71 per claim.[2] During the Demonstration period, the FI processed over 31,000 claims for children at the Comparison site at a cost of $202,018.

Administering the CHAMPUS system, however, also involved other costs. Since 1990, Health Management Strategies International, Inc. (HMS), has performed the precertification and continuing care reviews that CHAMPUS requires. HMS charged CHAMPUS $2.10 per eligible beneficiary. (This was the rate in the original 1990 contract. We inflated this rate using the consumer price index for medical care to create a rate for each year of the Demonstration.) The total cost of these services was $308,396.

Together, adding the costs of administering CHAMPUS to total expenditures at the Comparison site raises those costs to $14,144,163 and lowers the between-site difference by .93% to $32,774,648.

A second adjustment involves the costs of services provided by CHAMPUS to children in the Fort Bragg catchment area during the Demonstration period. This involved 1165 children, 569 of whom also received services at the Rumbaugh Clinic. Including the costs of processing the claims involved, expenditures on these services totaled $1,068,325. It is not clear how clients received these services. All providers in the area were informed that potential clients should be screened by the Rumbaugh Clinic, but the FI was permitted to pay claims for services provided. One could argue that a fair between-site comparison requires that all expenditures on children in each catchment area be included. In that case, these costs should be added to the costs of the Demonstration. Doing so raises total expenditures at the Demonstration site to $47,987,136.

---

[2]The actual number of claims and the processing charge per claim were as follows:

Fiscal year	Claims	$/Claim
1991	12,274	$6.56
1992	9,136	$6.71
1993	9,901	$6.08
1994	1,313	$6.08

Table 7.2. Estimated Adjustments in Total Costs for the Demonstration Period[a]

Cost component	Demonstration site		Comparison site		Cumulative between-site difference
	Adjustment	Cumulative adjusted total costs[b]	Adjustment	Cumulative adjusted total costs[b]	
Unadjusted estimates (from Table 7.1)	—	$46,918,811	—	$13,633,749	$33,285,062
FI costs associated with processing these claims	—	46,918,811	$202,018	13,835,767	33,083,044
HMS costs associated with running CHAMPUS	—	46,918,811	308,396	14,144,163	32,774,648
Services delivered by CHAMPUS in the Fort Bragg catchment area					
Children served by the Rumbaugh Clinic	$ 405,242	47,324,053	—	14,144,163	33,179,890
Children not served by the Rumbaugh Clinic	631,358	47,955,411	—	14,144,163	33,811,248
FI costs associated with these claims	31,725	47,987,136	—	14,144,163	33,842,973
Services delivered under Gateway	—	47,987,136	885,800	15,029,963	32,957,173
Costs related to the Demonstration (3%)	$1,407,564	$49,394,700	—	$15,029,963	$34,364,737

[a]These data describe the treated population at the Demonstration and Comparison sites. The Demonstration period is the combined fiscal years 1991–1993.
[b]The entries is these columns are accumulative totals of the unadjusted costs presented in Table 7.1 (and transferred as the entries in the first row of this table) and each necessary adjustment.

A third adjustment involves the costs of services delivered under Gateway. As discussed earlier, only outpatient services were provided on post under Gateway. A crude MIS provided by Fort Campbell represents the only source of information on these services. These data suggest that 4429 outpatient visits were delivered in fiscal years 1991, 1992, and 1993. If these services are valued at $100 per visit (the cost of outpatient services at the Demonstration site), it appears that services provided under Gateway were worth $442,900. Under the rather strong assumption that Gateway delivered a similar volume of services at Fort Stewart (and none at the Demonstration site), a total of $885,800 in services is added to total expenditures at the Comparison site. This addition raises total expenditures at the Comparison site to $15,029,963. It narrows the between-site gap in expenditures to $32,957,173.

A fourth and final adjustment involves the costs of managing a Demonstration. The budget figures on which the per-unit costs used to calculate Table 7.1 were based included only 97% of actual expenditures; 3% of expenditures was deducted as an adjustment for costs associated with administrating a Demonstration. This decision was an arbitrary one made by the administrators of the Rumbaugh Clinic. Adding these costs back in inflates all costs by 3% and raises the costs of the Demonstration to $49,394,699.

The combined effect of all four adjustments is modest: They raise the between-site difference to $34,364,736, a figure barely 3% higher than the unadjusted difference. This increase is entirely due to adding the estimated costs of running a demonstration back into the total costs of the Demonstration. The other three adjustments virtually negate each other.

QUESTION 2. DID THE DISTRIBUTION OF EXPENDITURES ACROSS CHILDREN AND SERVICES DIFFER BETWEEN SITES?

Table 7.3 documents the distribution of expenditures across major types of services. Differences in these distributions reflect the differences in utilization presented in Chapter 5. As the program theory would suggest, treatment in hospitals and residential treatment centers (RTCs) accounted for over 80% of total expenditures at the Comparison site, but only 25% at the Demonstration site. Expenditures at the Demonstration site were primarily for outpatient therapy and intermediate services. By themselves, both residential and nonresidential intermediate services accounted for as large a proportion of total expenditures as did hospitalization.

Table 7.3. Distribution of Costs per Treated Child by Service Type across Service Types and Costs[a]

Service	Demonstration site				Comparison site			
	Total	Proportion of total	Per child receiving the service	Per treated child	Total	Proportion of total	Per child receiving the service	Per treated child
Hospital	$11,075,509	23.65%	$22,107	$1,836	$ 6,424,853	47.74%	$16,224	$2,311
RTC	2,360,791	5.03%	33,726	391	4,703,437	34.95%	51,686	1,692
Intermediate residential	9,150,773	19.54%	26,835	1,517	Services not available at the Comparison sites			
Intermediate nonresidential	8,451,128	18.04%	17,073	1,401				
Outpatient	12,972,106	27.70%	2,471	2,150	1,765,325	13.12%	731	635
Assessment and evaluation	1,839,499	3.93%	334	305	563,665	4.19%	367	203
Case management	572,866	1.22%	427	95	Services not available at Comparison sites			
Treatment team	412,967	0.88%	80	68				
Total service costs	$46,835,659				$13,457,280			
Other costs[b]	83,172				176,469			
Total for Demonstration period[b]	$46,918,811	100.00%	—	7,777	$13,633,749	100.00%	—	$4,904

[a]These data describe the treated population at the Demonstration and Comparison sites. The Demonstration period is the combined fiscal years 1991–1993. The left column represents the type of service provided. Each entry in "Total" column is the total expenditure for the specified category of service. The "Proportion of total" column is the proportion of total costs that the type of service represents. The "Cost per child receiving the service" is the total expenditures on that service divided by the number of children receiving that service. The number of observations used to create this mean is the number of children receiving the specific category of services, taken from Table 5.4. The "Cost per treated child" represents total expenditures on the service divided by the number of children receiving *any* service of *any* type.

[b]The total costs for all services include costs of "other" services totaling $83,172 for the Demonstration site and $176,469 for the Comparison site. "Other costs" included procedures that were vague or not easily grouped into the defined service categories.

As discussed earlier, average expenditures per treated child were much higher at the Demonstration site. Averaging across treated children, however, obscures rather substantial variation in expenditures on each child. Table 7.4 presents expenditures on all children treated during the Demonstration period, grouping them by the amount spent on their care. Presented are the number of children in each category, the percentage of treated children that number represents, the percentage of total expenditures devoted to those children, and mean expenditures for children in that group.

Table 7.4 demonstrates how widely expenditures vary across individual children. At the Demonstration site, nearly one fourth of all children treated had expenditures below $500. Despite the size of this group, it accounted for less than 1% of expenditures. In contrast, the 7% of children with expenditures in excess of $25,000 accounted for over 70% of total expenditures.

The figures for the Comparison site reveal rather striking differences. Over half of all children treated at the Comparison site received less than $500 worth of services; this proportion is twice that for the Demonstration site. Children in this low-expenditure category had costs roughly half those at the Demonstration site. Thus, low-cost clients at the Comparison site had expenditures even lower than their counterparts at the Demonstration site. Likewise, a child treated at the Comparison site was significantly less likely to have expenditures exceeding $25,000. Of those with expenditures above that amount, individuals at the Demonstration site

Table 7.4. Distribution of Costs by Cost Category
for the Demonstration Period[a]

	Demonstration site				Comparison site			
Cost range	N	%	% of costs	Mean	N	%	% of costs	Mean
<$500	1411	23.39%	0.93%	$ 310	1502	54.03%	2.02%	$ 183
$500–$1000	1216	20.16%	1.91%	736	429	15.43%	2.22%	706
$1000–$2500	1630	27.02%	5.56%	1,601	319	11.47%	3.56%	1,523
$2500–$5,000	815	13.51%	6.01%	3,462	108	3.88%	2.71%	3,417
$5,000–$15,000	459	7.61%	7.93%	8,108	159	5.72%	10.59%	9,077
$15,000–$25,000	105	1.74%	4.37%	19,506	114	4.10%	16.38%	19,595
$25,000+	397	6.58%	73.29%	86,611	149	5.36%	62.52%	57,206
	6033	100.00%	100.00%		2780	100.00%	100.00%	

[a]These data describe the treated population at the Demonstration and Comparison sites. The Demonstration period is the combined fiscal years 1991–1993. The "N" column is the frequency distribution of the number of cases for the different ranges of costs (e.g., 1411 cases cost less than $500 at the Demonstration site). The "%" column is the percentage of all cases in each range. The "% of Costs" column is the percentage of total costs devoted to children in each range.

had much higher costs on average than their counterparts at the Comparison site.

QUESTION 3. WHAT EXPLAINS THE DIFFERENCE
IN SYSTEM-LEVEL COSTS?

Total expenditures may differ between sites for either of two reasons: More children were treated or expenditures were higher on each child treated. This section considers the relative importance of each.

Large increases in the number of children treated had a strong effect on system costs: It explains the majority of the cost increase at the Demonstration site. Had the average cost per client remained constant (at its 1988 level), costs in fiscal year 1993 would have risen to $14,631,059, over four fifths of the observed value for fiscal year 1993 ($17,365,676). Increased access, therefore, explains over 70% of the increase between fiscal year 1988 and fiscal year 1993 at the Demonstration site. The remaining 30% of the increase reflects differences in the costs of treating the average child. The difference over time includes the effect of inflation, which is assumed to be the same between sites.

Increased access cannot explain all the increase in expenditures—more money was spent on each child treated. Average expenditures per child increased by 25% (relative to historical levels) in the Fort Bragg catchment area. Had the Demonstration site been able to treat the 6033 children it treated at the average cost incurred at the Comparison site ($4904), total spending at the Demonstration site would have been just under $30 million. This suggests that roughly half of the between-site difference is due to increased access.[3]

The cost implications of the continuum of care largely concern the expenditures that would result from moving a child into a system conforming to its principles from one that did not. Understanding and interpreting the difference in average expenditures per treated child, therefore, seems especially important. Questions 4 and 5 examine the between-site difference in average expenditures per child more closely.

QUESTION 4. WHY DO AVERAGE EXPENDITURES
PER TREATED CHILD DIFFER?

The costs of treating the average child at the Demonstration site were higher for four reasons: longer time spent in treatment, greater volume of

---

[3]The difference in the two comparisons is that the increase in the number of children served was greater when measured against historical levels at Fort Bragg.

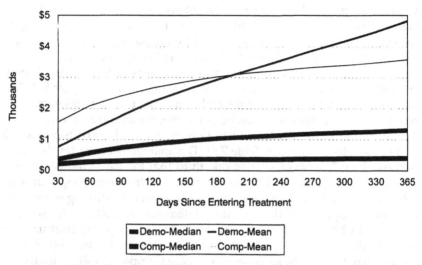

Figure 7.2. Median and mean costs by time since the child entered treatment.

traditional services, heavy use of intermediate services, and higher per-unit costs.

As discussed in Chapter 5, children at the Demonstration site stayed in treatment longer, and this is the first reason the costs of treating the average child was higher at the Demonstration site. This increased duration of treatment had striking implications for median costs of treating children. Figure 7.2 plots the mean and median costs for 30-day intervals over the first 365 days after the child entered treatment.[4] The median line for the Comparison site is flat, the reason being that after 180 days, the majority of children at the Comparison site were no longer in treatment. In contrast, the majority of children at the Demonstration site were still receiving services after 180 days. Consequently, the median cost for the Demonstration site continued to rise. The continued treatment of children at the Demonstration site beyond 180 days drives the site medians apart and accounted for some of the higher treatment costs at the Demonstration.

Mean costs, as presented in Figure 7.2, provide added insight. For the first 90 days children were in treatment, the Demonstration site was actually less expensive than the Comparison site; at 180 days, the means were

[4]As discussed earlier, for some children, this time period may be from the time the child entered the catchment area.

virtually identical. After 1 year in treatment, however, mean cost at the Demonstration site was much higher than at the Comparison site. Again, the reason for this difference is that children remained in treatment much longer at the Demonstration site than at the Comparison site.

A second explanation for the increased costs of treating the typical child at the Demonstration site was also highlighted in Chapter 5. When receiving services of a given type, children at the Demonstration site also received more of those services. For example, the average child receiving outpatient therapy at the Demonstration site received nearly $2500 worth of those services alone (see Table 7.3). The analogous figure for the Comparison site ($731) was less than one third that for the Demonstration.

The implications of children remaining in treatment longer and receiving more services of a given type were especially striking when only the costs of outpatient therapy, hospitalization, and RTCs (the services common to both sites) were examined. The average expenditure per treated child for these services at the Demonstration site was $4696, only 4% less than that for the same services at the Comparison site. Children at the Demonstration site received new services, but their use of traditional services was reduced only slightly.

The Demonstration made heavy use of intermediate services, and this heavier usage represents a third reason for the higher costs per treated child at the Demonstration site. Both the amount spent on intermediate residential and that spent on intermediate nonresidential services per treated client ($1517 and $1401) were higher than the amount spent on hospitalization [$1836 (see Table 7.3)]. The average child who received services in an intermediate residential setting received over $27,000 worth of that service.

It is worthwhile to note what did *not* substantially inflate costs at the Demonstration site. While virtually all children at the Demonstration site received the attention of treatment teams and many children received clinical case management, these services were fairly inexpensive (Table 7.3). They accounted for barely 2% of total spending at the Demonstration site and amounted to less than $200 per treated child.

A fourth and final reason that costs per treated child were higher at the Demonstration site is that costs per service were higher as well. Table 7.5 shows that the average cost of an outpatient service was 24% higher at the Demonstration site than at the Comparison site. There were similar differences for other services offered at both sites; hospitalization unit costs were 20% higher at the Demonstration site, and care in an RTC was 25% more costly at the Demonstration site.

What explains the higher per-unit costs at the Demonstration site? For hospitalization and RTC treatment, the Demonstration site may have used

Table 7.5. Per-Unit Charges for Each Service Category by Site for the Demonstration Period[a]

Service	Site	
	Demonstration	Comparison
Hospital	$584.08	$488.31
Residential treatment center	462.52	369.71
Intermediate residential	209.81	NA
Intermediate nonresidential	290.81	NA
Clinical case management	52.91	NA
Outpatient therapy	101.43	81.85
Assessment/evaluation	161.61	197.60
Treatment team services	49.88	NA

[a]These data describe the treated population at the Demonstration and Comparison sites. The Demonstration period is the combined fiscal years 1991–1993.

higher-cost providers.[5] Differences in per-unit costs for services (e.g., outpatient therapy) may also reflect hidden differences in utilization. As discussed in Chapter 2, we collapsed services of a given type on a given day into a single unit. The cost for this single unit of service reflects the total volume of services delivered. Higher per-unit costs at the Demonstration site may reflect the greater use of services on any given day where children received services of a given type. Thus, costs per service encounter may be higher at the Demonstration site even though the Rumbaugh Clinic may have contracted for external services at rates lower than the CHAMPUS rates presented. For example, the Pioneer per-unit cost for outpatient therapy was $85.64 for fiscal year 1993, an amount comparable to the CHAMPUS rate. Combining outpatient services that occurred on the same day, however, produced the higher rate in Table 7.5.

An alternative explanation of the site difference in outpatient per-unit costs may be that bookkeeping procedures on which per-unit costs were based were flawed. As discussed in Chapter 2, per-unit costs for all services were inflated by 16.8% to account for administrative overhead. If the actual administrative cost of outpatient therapy was lower than 16.8%, its cost was inflated. At most, however, this adjustment would explain only 16.8% of the difference in costs and cannot account completely for differ-

[5]This difference may be a function of the type of children sent to these facilities. As hospitalization was used less frequently, for example, it may have been reserved for the most severe children.

ences in outpatient costs. (If all overhead assigned was inappropriate, per-unit costs would have been 16.8% lower.)

Average expenditures per client were clearly higher at the Demonstration site, and this difference is largely a function of the fact that children treated there received more services. Does this mean that moving a child from the Comparison site to the Demonstration site would increase the services that child received and thus inflate expenditures on that child? Answering this question requires a more detailed examination of the effect of increased access on the mix of children receiving care and on the link between severity and service utilization.

QUESTION 5. WERE INTERMEDIATE SERVICES SUBSTITUTED FOR MORE EXPENSIVE AND RESTRICTIVE SERVICES?

Its proponents claim that one of the ways the continuum of care saves money is that it substitutes cheaper, less restrictive services for hospitalization. The figures in Table 7.5 appear to support this proposition: Clearly, on a per-day basis, intermediate services were considerably less expensive than inpatient hospitalization or care in an RTC.

For expenditures to be reduced, however, intermediate services have to be substituted for more restrictive services and not used to supplement those services. In addition, this substitution needs to be on a two-for-one basis (or less) (based on data in Table 7.5). Obviously, for example, if a day of hospitalization is replaced by 10 days of care in a group home, expenditures will increase, not decrease.

The Project assessed the effects of intermediate services on costs by comparing children who received those services with comparable children at the Comparison site. (A simple comparison of children at the Demonstration site who did and did not receive intermediate services would be misleading; it would ignore systematic differences between the two groups.)

Children at the Comparison site most like children receiving intermediate services at the Demonstration site were identified in a two-step procedure. First, a model predicting the use of intermediate services at the Demonstration site was estimated; this model identified the predictors of intermediate service use. Second, this model was used to estimate the likelihood that each child at the Comparison site would have received intermediate services had he or she been treated at the Demonstration site. Those children most likely to have received intermediate services form the comparison group in this analysis. (This procedure is described in more detail in Chapter 6.)

The last line of Table 7.6 presents mean and median costs for children who received intermediate services at the Demonstration site and for their predicted counterparts at the Comparison site. It can be seen that mean expenditures were nearly double; median expenditures for intermediate services were 5 times as high. Either because intermediate services did not reduce the use of hospitalization or because large volumes of intermediate services were used, the use of intermediate services did not reduce expenditures.

QUESTION 6. ARE THE DIFFERENCES IN AVERAGE EXPENDITURES PER TREATED CHILD DUE TO DIFFERENCES IN THE MIX OF CHILDREN TREATED?

The preceding discussion has treated differences in access and in expenditures per child as distinct determinants of between-site differences in costs. The two, however, are related. Expenditures per treated child represent expenditures on the typical child, and the level of access to services will influence the type of children receiving services.

The potential effects of access on the mix of children receiving services can have a dramatic impact on how differences in service utilization—and, by extension, costs—are interpreted. The use of intermediate services, for example, may have been high at the Demonstration site *not* because these services were lavished on children already receiving care, but because new children entered the system and received the new services. Fewer than 900 children received intermediate services during the entire Demonstration period, while the number of children served in a given fiscal year increased by more than 2000 children. The large increase in access, therefore, may have altered the mix of children at the Demonstration site, so that the "typical" child there differed from the "typical" child at the Comparison site. This possibility is especially important if the Demonstration site drew children of higher severity into the system. In this case, the Demonstration was more costly not because it treated children differently but because it treated different children.

Accounting for differences in the pool of clients requires a means of controlling for client severity. The Project did so by comparing children with similar scores on an index of severity (refer to Chapter 5 for a discussion of the severity measure). The first three rows in Table 7.6 show the mean costs per child by severity. As expected, costs increased with severity. At all levels, mean costs were higher at the Demonstration site:

Table 7.6. Mean and Median Costs for the Demonstration Period
by Severity for the Evaluation Sample[a]

Severity	Demonstration site			Comparison site			Ratio of demonstration site to comparison site	
	N	Median	Mean	N	Median	Mean	Median	Mean
Level of severity								
High	144	$13,924	$24,605	102	$7,519	$14,798	1.85	1.66[b]
Moderate	279	1,572	8,513	210	1,256	5,798	1.25	1.47[b]
Low	151	1,207	4,516	93	789	1,870	1.53[b]	2.42[b]
Received intermediate services	70	17,047	22,715	92	3,197	13,571	5.33[b]	1.65[b]

[a]These data describe the experiences of the Evaluation Sample between Waves 1 and 2 of the Demonstration period. The last row, "Received intermediate services," presents the median and mean costs for children receiving those services. The Comparison site did not offer these services, but an algorithm based on the characteristics of Demonstration children receiving intermediate services was used to predict which children at the Comparison sites would have received them had they been at the Demonstration site.
[b]Between-site difference significant at $p < 0.05$.

2.42, 1.47, and 1.66 times as expensive for children of low, moderate, and high severity, respectively. (Median costs were consistent with these results.)

These comparisons suggest that average costs per client were high at the Demonstration site not simply because the pool of treated children changed. Rather, expenditures on children of comparable severity were higher at the Demonstration site. This finding suggests that moving a child from the Comparison site to the Demonstration site would have increased expenditures on that child.

QUESTION 7. HOW DID THE DEMONSTRATION AFFECT COSTS OUTSIDE THE SPECIALTY MENTAL HEALTH SECTOR?

It appears that—in terms of direct expenditures on specialty mental health services—the Demonstration was more costly. It is unclear, however, whether these costs were offset by reduced costs elsewhere. This acknowledgment is especially important in light of the limitations of our data. As discussed earlier, we lack comprehensive data on costs in other systems (such as juvenile justice) and on the costs associated with untreated children. We can fill in the blanks somewhat, however, using supplemental data. These data come from two sources: reports by parents in the Evaluation Sample and data on children in State facilities in the State of Tennessee.

Caretakers of children in the Evaluation Sample reported on the following costs associated with their children's illness: travel costs associated with obtaining treatment, damage to property and injuries sustained or inflicted by the child, parental employment problems resulting from the child's disorder, and care children received outside the specialty mental health sector. These reports all describe the 6-month period between Waves 1 and 2 of data collection. We analyzed these reports and measured the costs associated with the outcomes reported. Between-site cost differences were then adjusted to account for these differences.

Tables 7.7–7.9 present the results of these analyses. Table 7.7 describes the transportation costs related to treatment. These costs involve the out-of-pocket expenses (such as gasoline) as well as time lost traveling. We present these results for each severity category so that our comparisons involve children of comparable severity. As expected, parents of more severe children traveled farther and thus spent more time in transit. Caretakers of the most severely impaired children at the Demonstration site reported traveling an average of 922 miles during the 6-month period. This distance was triple that traveled by parents of the least severe children (304

Table 7.7. Adjusted Transportation Costs by Severity[a]

Severity	Cost	Demonstration site				Comparison site				Between-site difference	p-value[b]
		Mean	Value	Cases	Cumulative costs	Mean	Value	Cases	Cumulative costs		
Least	Unadjusted figure	—	—		$ 4,516	—	—		$ 1,870	$2,646	—
	Miles traveled	304.27	$ 76	97	4,592	321.56	$ 80	66	1,950	2,775	90%
	Hours traveling	22.88	204	103	4,796	7.32	65	68	2,015	2,918	<1%
Moderate	Unadjusted figure	—			8,516	—			5,798	2,718	
	Miles traveled	479.66	120	182	8,636	270.90	68	152	5,866	2,770	2%
	Hours traveling	32.04	285	196	8,921	25.96	231	149	6,097	2,824	12%
Most	Unadjusted figure	—			24,608	—			14,798	9,810	—
	Miles traveled	922.41	231	94	24,839	1120.20	280	73	15,078	9,761	46%
	Hours traveling	45.67	406	98	25,245	42.75	380	80	15,458	9,787	73%

[a]These data describe the experiences of the Evaluation Sample between Waves 1 and 2 of the Demonstration period. The entries in the "Value" column are the products of miles traveled or hours traveling and the value of a mile traveled ($0.25) or an hour of work (at the average wage for the entire Evaluation Sample of $8.90/hour). The entries in the "Cumulative cost" column are cumulative totals for each severity level accounting for each travel cost adjustment.
[b]For a t-test of between-site differences in the mean number of miles traveled or hours spent traveling.

miles). A similar link exists between severity and time spent in transit. Caretakers of the most severely impaired children at the Demonstration site reported having spent an average of 46 hours in treatment-related travel during the previous 6 months. This travel time was twice the time for caretakers of the least severely impaired. The relationship between treatment-related travel and severity holds at the Comparison site as well.

Treatment-related transportation can be expressed in monetary terms. Mileage costs were valued at $.25/mile; travel time was valued at the mean wage of the primaray caretaker ($8.90/hour). With respect to transportation costs, only two significant differences were detected: hours traveling for the least severe children, and miles of travel for the moderately severe. In both instances, the service system at the Demonstration site proved to be more costly: on average, travel time for the least severe cost $139 more; parents of moderately severe children at the Demonstration site parents paid an additional $52 in transportation costs. Thus, factoring in transportation costs serves only to widen the between-site differences in average cost per treated child.

Reports from caretakers of children in the Evaluation Sample included information on damage and injuries for which sample members were responsible. Table 7.8 shows that between-site differences in these costs were generally insignificant. Children of moderate severity at the Demonstration site were more likely, however, to have injured themselves or others (not presented in this table).

Table 7.8 also presents parental reports of employment difficulties that caretakers experienced as a result of a child's problems. Also reported are

Table 7.8. Supplemental Costs of Mental Disorders
by Site for the Evaluation Sample[a]

Experience during the past 6 months	Cases	Demonstration	Comparison	$p(\chi^2)$
Parent had employment problems as a result of the child's problems.	819	44.41%	42.95%	0.68
Family members (other than the child) missed school as a result of the child's problems.	775	11.85%	10.76%	0.63
Child destroyed property.	781	22.22%	18.75%	0.23
Child injured someone (including himself or herself).	772	13.64%	17.42%	0.15

[a]These data describe the experiences of the Evaluation Sample between Waves 1 and 2 of the Demonstration period.

any school problems other members of the family experienced. Again, the likelihood that such problems occurred increased dramatically as the severity of the child's problems increased, but the differences between sites were not statistically significant.

Table 7.9 summarizes parental reports of services that children in the Evaluation Sample received outside the specialty mental health sector. The parent was asked about a wide range of services. The table reports the mean number of contacts per child, disaggregated by severity. The pattern for these services was the same as for the indirect costs examined above; more severe cases used these services more frequently. However, there was only one statistically significant difference between the sites: Children with the least severe problems at the Demonstration site were more likely to call a crisis hotline than their counterparts at the Comparison site.

The use of services outside the specialty mental health sector did not vary by site. Regardless of their costs, therefore, incorporating them into the cost analysis could not influence the relative costliness of the Demonstration. A second source of data, however, provided information of potentially greater impact. In Tennessee, children in State custody could receive care in a private psychiatric hospital or in a residential treatment center. If access to CHAMPUS-reimbursed services was denied on post or by HMS review, service providers or Army personnel sometimes encouraged parents to petition juvenile court for State custody. Note that this practice was not possible in Georgia or Kentucky (with the exception noted below).

Because Medicaid or State funds were used to pay for these services, they do not appear in CHAMPUS records. In fact, this practice reduced the costs of caring for CHAMPUS-eligible children in Tennessee. Because of the high quality of services available at the Demonstration site, similar children were treated at the site. The Demonstration site may appear more expensive not because children in the catchment area received more services but because it shifted fewer costs onto the State.

The key question involves the extent to which this practice occurred in Tennessee. The State of Tennessee provided fiscal year 1991 records for children in State custody. These records revealed that 23 children hospitalized or treated in RTCs at the State's expense were CHAMPUS-eligible. This treatment involved a total of 1305 hospital days and 1450 days in RTCs. Valuing these services at what they would have cost had they been provided through CHAMPUS raises the costs of caring for children at the Comparison site by $1,173,324 for fiscal year 1991.

Table 7.10 shows the effects of including the costs of treating these children on total costs, costs per treated child, and costs per eligible child. (Data were available only for fiscal year 1991, so we assumed that these

Table 7.9. Other Indirect Costs in the Evaluation Sample[a]

Experience during the past 6 months	Least severe		Moderately severe		Most severe	
	Demo (N)	Comp (N)	Demo (N)	Comp (N)	Demo (N)	Comp (N)
Damage and injuries (% reporting)	123	88	224	179	114	98
Damaged property	10%	9%	18%	20%	30%	38%
Injured self or others	9%	10%	19%	12%	24%	20%
Job or school difficulties (% reporting)						
Caretaker experienced employment difficulties	22%	26%	38%	35%	55%	49%
Other family members missed school	8%	6%	11%	12%	13%	18%
Other services (mean	119	82	217	168	112	86
number of days of contact or service)	(N)	(N)	(N)	(N)	(N)	(N)
Crisis hotline	0.03[b]	0.00	0.12	0.06	0.94	0.18
Religious figure	0.13	0.05	0.35	0.10	0.13	0.44
24-hour crisis center	0.21	0.00	0.01	0.01	0.08	0.00
Self-help group	0.31	0.00	0.21	0.45	2.56	3.17
Parent support group	0.35	0.18	0.25	1.10	1.35	0.57
School counselors	2.68	4.79	3.07	3.80	7.20	5.52
Enrolled in special class or school	3.38	4.89	4.51	4.41	8.83	18.44
Evaluation/testing agency	0.25	0.15	0.22	0.27	0.81	0.42
Advice/support						
Nonprofessional, nonfamily adult	0.60	0.55	1.20	1.95	3.11	2.21
Friends	4.85	5.91	4.79	7.14	12.24	9.52
Probation/law enforcement officer	0.08	0.41	0.16	0.35	0.58	0.47
Stay in detention center	0.01	0.07	0.21	0.08	0.13	3.82
Exceptional Family Member Program	0.07	0.15	0.90	2.10	5.05	4.86
Army Community Services	0.01	0.09	0.07	0.11	0.15	0.14

[a]These data describe the experiences of the Evaluation Sample between Waves 1 and 2 of the Demonstration period.
[b]$p < 0.05$.

Table 7.10. Adjusting Cost Figures for Children Treated in State Facilities

Fiscal year	Number treated	Proportion of eligible children treated	Total amount	Costs per child	Costs per eligible child
A. Fort Campbell					
1990	576	2.53%	$4,975,361	$8,638	$219
1991	628	2.51%	$2,766,187	$4,405	$110
1992	489	2.46%	$ 892,213	$1,825	$ 45
1993	404	1.87%	$ 772,574	$1,912	$ 36
B. Fort Stewart					
1990	666	3.36%	$3,647,713	$5,477	$184
1991	695	3.35%	$4,373,704	$6,293	$211
1992	619	3.46%	$2,455,610	$3,967	$137
1993	741	3.61%	$2,873,403	$3,878	$140
C. Fort Campbell with adjustment for Gateway and children in state custody					
1991	647	2.58%	$3,941,831	$6,092	$157
1992	1058	5.33%	$2,347,557	$2,219	$118
1993	986	4.57%	$2,170,878	$2,202	$101
D. Fort Stewart with adjustment for Gateway					
1992	952	5.33%	$2,540,505	$2,669	$142
1993	939	4.57%	$2,923,852	$3,114	$142

costs were constant over time.) Since children were treated under State custody only at Fort Campbell, costs for the two locations in the Comparison site are presented separately. Before considering the effect of care received by children in State custody, we first compare and contrast the two Comparison-sites locations.

The unadjusted figures for Fort Campbell (section A) and Fort Stewart (section B) show that costs per treated child and costs per eligible child fell at both Comparison-site locations throughout the early 1990s. Given the changes that were occurring in the military's health care system, this decline is hardly surprising. As medical expenditures increased nationwide, spending for mental health services for military dependents decreased rather dramatically. Wojcik, Stein, and Optenberg (1993) reported that in the typical Health Services Command catchment area, mental health expenditures per eligible dependent under the age of 18 fell by nearly 30% between 1990 and 1992.[6]

It is also clear from Table 7.10, however, that cost reductions at the

[6]Wojcik et al. (1993) report median monthly expenditures per 1000 eligible dependents for the month of June. These figures seem to suggest a rate of change roughly comparable to those reported here. For example, Table 7.10 suggests that expenditures per eligible fell by 136% at Fort Campbell; Wojcik et al. (1993) report a 160% decrease. No doubt the changes reported reflect changes in access, but Wojcik et al. (1993) do not report costs per treated child and were unable to provide this information to us.

combined Comparison-site locations reported above were driven largely by changes at Fort Campbell. The reductions at Fort Campbell were much larger than at Fort Stewart and at other posts across the country. Wojcik et al. (1993) ranked all catchment areas according to the amount by which expenditures per eligible child fell. Of the 36 catchment areas, Fort Campbell led the nation; Its decrease between fiscal year 1990 and fiscal year 1992 (−160%) was 7 times the rate of decline at the typical (median) post (−23%). Fort Stewart, however, was far more representative. Average expenditures per eligible child there fell by 16%, an amount somewhat less than the typical (median) post.

What effect does incorporating the costs of care children received in State custody have on differences between the two Comparison-site locations and on the two locations when combined? Sections C and D of Table 7.10 show the effect these costs have on access, total costs, costs per child, and costs per eligible child. Note that the adjusted figures for Fort Campbell (section C) include both the costs of care received by children in State custody and the costs associated with the Gateway to Care system discussed above.

Section C presents the revised figures for Fort Campbell. Incorporating services received outside CHAMPUS raised the percentage of eligible children treated and the cost per eligible child significantly. CHAMPUS figures alone suggested that 1.87% of all children in the catchment area were treated in fiscal year 1993. Incorporating the supplemental information, however, raised this percentage to 4.57%. Obviously, the increase in access is due to Gateway, not to the small number of children supported by the State of Tennessee. Incorporating data on children treated under Gateway and on children in State custody raised the cost per treated child from $1912 to $2202 (fiscal year 1993). This increase was due to the addition of costs of treating children in State custody; including clients treated under Gateway actually reduced costs per treated child. These adjustments increased costs per eligible child rather dramatically as well. In fiscal year 1993, for example, CHAMPUS expenditures per eligible child totaled only $36; adding the costs of services under Gateway and to children in State custody increased costs per eligible child threefold, to $101.

Section D presents adjusted figures for Fort Stewart. Because CHAMPUS-eligible children could not receive care in State custody in Georgia, these adjustments reflect the effect of Gateway only. Lacking an MIS describing the services provided by Gateway at Fort Stewart, we examined potential effects by assuming that Gateway functioned the same way at Fort Campbell and Fort Stewart: We assumed that the percentage of eligible children served at Fort Stewart equaled that at Fort Campbell. It was also assumed that a child receiving services at Fort Stewart received the same amount of services (roughly $255 per fiscal year). Thus, we assumed that in fiscal year 1992, Gateway served 333 additional children, at a cost of $84,895. For fiscal year 1993, the figures were 198 children and $50,449.

In sum, while the costs of services received by children in State custody was rather substantial in absolute terms, it did not dramatically alter the gap in total costs between the Demonstration site and the Comparison site. Higher expenditures at the Demonstration site were not offset by reduced public expenditures on children in State custody.

SUMMARY OF COST FINDINGS

This chapter examined expenditures on mental health services under a continuum of care. It did so at both the system level (total costs) and the individual level (cost per treated child); at both levels, the continuum of care was more expensive. Within the limitations noted, it appears that these costs were not offset by cost savings elsewhere.

At the system level, instituting a continuum of care increased mental health expenditures for the Army relative to those under the usual CHAMPUS system. The Demonstration site was 3.29 times more expensive per eligible child. To a large extent, this increase reflected greater access to services. Nonetheless, costs per treated child were considerably higher at the Demonstration site. These higher costs reflect the fact that clients at the Demonstration site used more services and remained in treatment longer.

A key premise of the continuum-of-care treatment paradigm is that making less restrictive services available will decrease mental health care costs. Comparisons of children who received intermediate services with comparable children revealed that the introduction of intermediate services will not necessarily reduce expenditures.

Analyses of data from the Evaluation Sample and from the State of Tennessee revealed that increased expenditures at the Demonstration site were not exclusively a function of cost shifting from other service sectors. Costs savings elsewhere were not nearly large enough to explain the large difference in expenditures between sites.

Note that these findings must be interpreted in the context of the financial arrangements under which the Rumbaugh Clinic operated. As discussed in Chapter 1, the Demonstration operated under a cost-reimbursement contract. It had little financial incentive to control costs. In fact, as traditional economic theory would predict, the Demonstration consistently exceeded its budgeted expenditures. In part, this overrun can be attributed to client flow that initially exceeded budget estimates. There was also some indication that the Rumbaugh Clinic's Utilization Review system was not fully operational during the period these findings represent (see Heflinger, 1993). In addition, because parents bore no financial burden, a second limitation on service use was removed. Whether this was desirable—or wasteful—can be interpreted only in light of changes in mental health outcomes.

8

Discussion and Implications

REVISITING THE PROGRAM THEORY

According to the program model presented throughout this volume and a final time in Figure 8.1, the Demonstration had to meet multiple assumptions to obtain the predicted outcomes. If any of these assumptions were not met, then the Demonstration would not produce the hypothesized ultimate effects:

- Improved mental health outcome
- Quicker recovery
- Lower costs per client
- Better client satisfaction

Since the program model was based on a system-level intervention, it is important to differentiate this level of intervention from a simpler, service-level intervention. A system-level evaluation is concerned with the effectiveness of the organization and delivery of services, in contrast to the examination of the effectiveness of particular service components. It is the complex package of services at the Demonstration site that was being evaluated, not individual service components (such as psychotherapy or case management).

The system-level theory could be valid (i.e., the continuum of care could be better) and the Demonstration might still not be shown to be more effective unless four conditions were met:

- The system-level theory had to be well implemented (i.e., the continuum of care had to be well implemented at the Demonstration site).

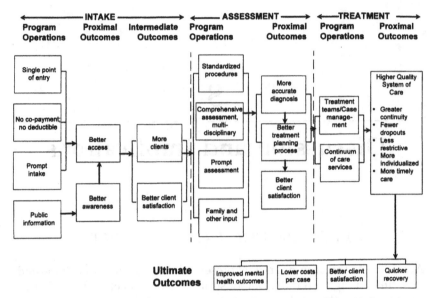

Figure 8.1. Fort Bragg Child and Adolescent Demonstration: Program theory.

- The service-level theory had to be valid (i.e., the theory that clinical services can improve outcomes must be true).
- The services had to be well implemented (i.e., the clinical services had to be well implemented at the Demonstration site).
- The evaluation had to be well implemented (i.e., the evaluation had to be rigorously conducted).

The Demonstration site could not be shown to be more effective than the Comparison site if theory at either the system or service level was not well implemented. The system-level aspects of the Demonstration site included intake and assessment, case management, and the variety of services available for treating clients. The service-level aspects of the Demonstration were the direct mental health services provided to clients. The service-level theory would fail if such services were ineffective. Finally, theories could be correct and well implemented at both the system and service levels, but we could still have failed to detect positive outcomes if the evaluation was faulty. The next two sections focus on implementation issues at the system and service level, and the following section discusses the evaluation itself.

SYSTEM-LEVEL IMPLEMENTATION

The Demonstration had to put appropriate components of service in place and ensure that the components were well integrated. These services had to be available to clients in a timely manner to produce smooth transitions from one service level to another. In other words, the level of service needs of clients had to be carefully monitored, and changes in those needs should have been accommodated quickly. If the Demonstration did not implement these critical features of the theory, then this study would not be a valid test of the theory. Moreover, both services and their management had to be available and of sufficient quality (i.e., an excellent case-management system cannot affect clinical outcomes unless appropriate, direct mental health services are available to be managed). Demonstration management and staff were responsible for the appropriate implementation of the theory at the system level.

The Fort Bragg Evaluation was responsible for documenting the implementation of the theory, but could not judge the effectiveness of individual components of the Demonstration at the system level (e.g., intake and assessment, case management), since assignment of clients to those system components was not random, but systematic (as related to clients' needs). This mode of assignment was a significant limitation, since there are few scientifically valid studies demonstrating that any of the specific components at the system level (e.g., case management) have actually improved the mental health of clients, even when properly implemented.

The possibility of failure was assessed at the system level by several methods. A brief discussion of the analysis of the implementation of the Demonstration is provided. Next, findings concerning the measurement of the quality of two key system-level components are described. Finally, relevant service utilization data testing differences between the Demonstration and Comparison sites and program theory are summarized.

Implementation Analysis

Several steps were necessary to comprehensively evaluate the Demonstration model. The theories and assumptions underlying the intervention were explicated, as represented in Figure 8.1. The program-as-implemented was compared to the program-as-planned, and any structural, environmental, or political barriers to full-scale implementation of the program were documented.

The overall strategy for examining program implementation was based on the theory-driven and component approaches (Bickman, 1985, 1987, 1990; Chen, 1990; Chen & Rossi, 1983) to program evaluation. The evaluators nominated specific structural and procedural aspects of implementation for each of the major implementation questions. A case study approach (Yin, 1986, 1993) described the structure and processes of the Demonstration and focused on operations during the third year of the Demonstration (fiscal year 1992) as an example of the fully functioning system. This case study approach incorporated multiple methods and multiple sources of information. As a result, the Demonstration generated a wealth of documentation that was available for review and analysis, including correspondence, program descriptions, policies and procedures, administrative reports, and committee meeting minutes.

On the basis of data from the Implementation Study (see Heflinger, 1993), it was evident that the Demonstration had been implemented consistent with the expectations of the contract and program theory by implementing a single point of entry to services for the target population, meeting the terms of the contract regarding participant eligibility (i.e., age, beneficiary status, and diagnostic eligibility), and serving three times the number of children originally estimated. Clients served at the Demonstration site had similar clinical characteristics of at least the same severity as clients served through the Civilian Health and Medical Program of the Uniformed Services (CHAMPUS) at the Comparison site. Thus, the increased number of children served did not reflect families seeking "unnecessary" treatment, but rather indicated that many children had previously had difficulty accessing needed services. The continuum-of-care model proposed by the Demonstration was implemented according to the expectations of the contract and program service philosophy through the provision of a comprehensive range of services, including development of intermediate service levels (intensive outpatient and substance abuse services, in-home crisis stabilization, day treatment, therapeutic home services, and group home), case management and multidisciplinary treatment teams for clients in the most intensive levels of care, and a high level of coordination of mental health services throughout the community for military dependent children.

Additional findings of the Implementation Study indicated that qualified staff were recruited, hired, and trained, and a fully operational quality improvement system was implemented.

The effects of the Demonstration's community-level coordination of services to military dependent children in the Fort Bragg area included fewer reported system-level problems, greater adequacy and higher quality of mental health services, better service system performance, and better adherence to the goals of an ideal service system. In each of these areas, the effects on military dependent children increased over time and were significantly more positive at Fort Bragg than at the Comparison sites.

In conclusion, the Implementation Study not only provided a comprehensive description of how the Demonstration was put in place, but also concluded that the Demonstration was executed with sufficient fidelity to provide an excellent test of the program theory—the continuum of care.

Quality of System-Level Components

From the perspective of the Fort Bragg Evaluation, the Quality Study and the Implementation Study were critical not only in describing the substance of the Demonstration, but also in setting the stage for the subsequent Cost/Utilization and Outcome Studies. Evidence was needed that program theory had been implemented as planned at the system level and that key system-level service components were of sufficient quality to produce the theoretically predicted effect on mental health.

Quality of mental health services is complex to define (Bickman & Peterson, 1990; McGlynn, Norquist, Wells, Sullivan, & Lieberman, 1988; Peterson & Bickman, 1992; Wells, 1988). Mental health services have many components and dimensions, and generally the definition of quality is subjective (i.e., dependent upon the perspective of the individual, the health care provider, the payer, or, ultimately, society). Thus, it has been recognized that the definition of quality depends on who does the defining.

Previous research on mental health services often described services similar to a "black box," whereby "inputs" and "outcomes" were studied, but what took place inside the box (where actual treatment occurs) went unstudied. This study was an initial attempt to systematically represent some of the workings within the black box. The component theory of evaluation (Bickman, 1985) was developed as a comprehensive means of first describing and then assessing statewide services delivered to preschool children. The logic behind this approach was that evaluations could be designed to examine individual components of a program (or service) rather than the entire program or service. A component is viewed as the largest homogeneous unit of a service. Components, then, serve as the building blocks of services and, although not fully independent of one another, may be studied separately.

At the core of the component method is identification of critical components of a service or program, followed by prioritization of those components based on the judgments of experts. The resulting product is an inventory of key components. An advantage of the component approach is that it is in tune with a "continuous improvement" theory of quality (Berwick, 1990). Continuous improvement aims at working alongside providers to improve services. The component approach fits well, because it provides an evaluation of key components rather than of the service as a whole. This approach, then, avoids labeling an entire service as good or bad, and instead focuses on different aspects of different services.

The Quality Study (see Bickman et al., 1993) evaluated two service components unique and crucial to the continuum-of-care model: intake assessment and case management. These components were chosen as the foci for the Quality Study because they are defined, developed, and implemented differently in a continuum of care than in typical treatment settings. Furthermore, these two components were selected because they encompass the primary activities and philosophies of the program.

The instruments used to measure quality of services for the components were similar. They included an instrument that measured parental satisfaction with the intake assessment, treatment planning, and case management; a semistructured interview administered to staff members performing intake assessment that addressed background, job attitude, and perceptions of the intake process; a scale that examined philosophy of care administered to all Rumbaugh Clinic staff (the Community Program Philosophy Scale); a questionnaire administered to direct service providers outside the Rumbaugh Clinic about the quality of intake assessment at Rumbaugh Clinic; an activity log completed by case managers; an expert review of medical records; and a network analysis that examined interagency coordination of services and the impact of that coordination at both the Demonstration site and the Comparison site.

The results of the Quality Study showed that the intake and assessment component was of high quality. Parents were satisfied with the intake and assessment service they received, and staff members were pleased with their jobs. Providers outside the Clinic rated the Rumbaugh Clinic intake process as being of high quality. The expert reviewer was able to find documented evidence of quality indicators within the clinical records. Intake and assessment at the Demonstration site was rated as the highest in adequacy and quality of all the support services available.

The Quality data also illustrated a great deal of faithfulness on the part of intake and assessment staff to the indices of quality identified by the stakeholder groups, as well as the philosophy of the Demonstration.

Case management services at the Rumbaugh Clinic were exemplary for most of the clients, with a high degree of fidelity to the values of stakeholders. There was a strong emphasis on planning and coordination of the treatment plan, in keeping with the written expectations of the Army contract and the job description for case managers. Careful attention was paid to meeting standards for treatment reviews and level-of-care criteria. Generally positive satisfaction ratings by parents suggested that case management activities were carried out in a way that promoted client and family involvement.

Utilization of Services

While improving the quality of traditional services may have an effect on mental health outcomes, such an improvement was not the primary objective of the Demonstration. The key aspect of the theory of the Demonstration was the centralized management of traditional services plus provision of nontraditional services believed to be more appropriate for the client. These services included group homes, therapeutic homes, day treatment, and the availability of wraparound or other supportive services. The service utilization data presented in Chapter 4 indicated that children received services sooner, care was provided in less restrictive environments, there was heavy use of intermediate-level services, children stayed in treatment longer, length of stay was shorter in hospitals and residential treatment centers (RTCs), the number of readmissions to hospitals and RTCs was higher, and there were fewer disruptions in services and fewer clients who received only one session of outpatient treatment.

In summary, the Fort Bragg Demonstration was viewed as a very successful implementation of the continuum-of-care theory at the system level. Data from the Implementation and Quality Studies demonstrated that the model was implemented with great fidelity. Service utilization data indicated that access to care more than tripled and that children at similar levels of impairment were more likely to be treated without a hospital stay at the Demonstration site than were children at the Comparison site. These findings indicated that system implementation failure at the Demonstration site is unlikely to have occurred.

SERVICE-LEVEL THEORY AND IMPLEMENTATION

The next way the Demonstration could have appeared ineffective was if its clinical services were not effective. The Demonstration's staff and management could have faithfully and completely implemented all the system-level aspects of the theory, and we could still have shown that the Demonstration had no effect. This outcome would have been possible if the direct mental health services (e.g., psychotherapy, hospitalization) provided by the Demonstration were not effective in altering clients' mental health status. These components of services could have failed to be effective if they were, in fact, ineffective, or if the Demonstration did not implement them with sufficient quality. As with system-level components, few previous studies have demonstrated that psychotherapy with children is effective in community settings (Weisz & Weiss, 1993). Furthermore, there is no clear scientific evidence that the other forms of intervention

used in the Demonstration are efficacious (Rivera & Kutash, 1994), although this lack may be more a reflection of a lack of research studies than
evidence that the services are ineffective. It was possible, however, for the
Demonstration theory to be correct and the Demonstration to be adequately implemented at the system level, but for us to find no effects on
clients' mental health. That is, the Demonstration may have been very
effectively delivering seemingly appropriate and timely services, with
better continuity, that were nonetheless ineffective. Finally, the services
might have been theoretically effective, but the Demonstration may not
have delivered them with sufficient quality to have an effect on outcome.

The Demonstration was responsible for delivering what are believed
to be effective services. It was not responsible, however, for producing
positive outcomes even if those services are only believed to be, but in fact
are not, effective. As at the system level, we documented the Demonstration's implementation of the continuum-of-care theory and its proximal
effects on utilization, but were unable to judge the effectiveness of individual service components, since clients were not randomly assigned to individual components. We did find, however, that children at both sites
improved significantly. This improvement may be due to the treatment
provided at both sites.

Quality-Improvement Activities

To examine the effectiveness or quality of every direct component of
care in a continuum is impossible in any single study. As a pragmatic and
economical substitute for studying each component of care, however,
extant program resources can often be used to study service-level issues.
An assessment of the Demonstration's own quality improvement (QI)
activities in its evaluation provided needed information. According to
stipulations of the Army contract, the Demonstration had to follow the
requirements of the Joint Commission on Accreditation of Health Care
Organizations (JCAHO). Consistent with the JCAHO model (JCAHO,
1991, 1993), the Demonstration's QI was a complex management tool,
including credentialing and privileging of clinicians, monitoring against
indicators of quality programming, clinical care studies, and utilization
reviews. QI indicators were developed for each service component to
reflect issues of quality and to identify areas needing further investigation
through clinical care studies. Examples of such indicators are (in emergency services) the number of clients moving from telephone interview to
face-to-face interview to hospital admission per month and (in diagnostic
services) the number of days elapsing between the family's request for
services and the scheduled intake assessment. Essentially, in areas in
which the Demonstration planned to implement QI activities, the extent to

which the Demonstration met its own QI criteria and standards was assessed. These efforts were supplemented by a consultant who had extensive experience in this area.

The consultant's report indicated that the Rumbaugh Clinic's QI program complied, in both design and implementation, with JCAHO standards, especially concerning evaluation and monitoring of services. Moreover, it was noted that staff used the data generated by QI activities to improve program elements.[1] In general, the consultant had high praise for the QI program at the Rumbaugh Clinic. Furthermore, these findings were supported by Army Health Services Command reviewers of the QI program (Flannery, 1992). It was assumed that a well-designed and well-implemented QI program would help assure that direct services were also well implemented. Given the data from the Implementation and Quality Studies, this assumption appears to have been reasonable.

EVALUATION ISSUES

Finally, the Demonstration may have been properly implemented at both the system and the service level, and the services may have been effective and well implemented. Thus, children may have actually changed for the better while the Project failed to uncover these changes. Failure of any evaluation can be categorized into four types of concerns (Hedrick, Bickman, & Rog, 1993): (1) statistical validity—the extent to which the study has used the appropriate design and statistical methods to enable it to detect the effects that are present; (2) internal validity—the extent to which causal conclusions can be drawn between the program and the predicted outcomes; (3) construct validity—the extent to which the constructs in the conceptual framework are operationalized successfully (e.g., measured) in the research study; and (4) external validity—the extent to which it is possible to generalize from the data and context of the research study to broader populations and settings (especially those specified in the statement of the original problem or issue).

Statistical Validity

Initial Statistical Power

The statistical power (i.e., the ability of an evaluation to detect an effect that is really there) of any research design is critical. In a review of a

---

[1]This use of QI data should not be confused with the discussion in Chapter 5, which noted that cost data from the Rumbaugh Clinic's Utilization Review and Utilization Management Plan were not adequately incorporated into treatment decisions.

large number of meta-analyses of various interventions, Lipsey, Crosse Dunkle, Pollard, and Stobart (1985) found that published studies had les than a 50–50 chance of detecting an effect that was really there. That is, ar underpowered design would result in a finding of "no difference" when in fact, there was a difference between the treatment and control groups Several factors contribute to the power of the design, including th strength and integrity of the intervention, the sensitivity of the instrument used to measure outcomes, and the statistical analysis used. However, th clearest and most easily measured variable that contributes to statistica power is sample size.

From the initial planning of the Project, a sufficiently large sample to detect an effect size of clinical importance was required. As more informa tion about both the characteristics of the Project instruments and attritior became available, an empirical estimate of power based on Monte Carl modeling (Lambert, 1993) was produced that provided an estimate of th number of clients (950 participants) needed for the study. As noted ii Chapter 2, a great deal of effort was expended to recruit an initial sample o sufficient size to detect meaningful effects.

Attrition

In a longitudinal study, two factors contribute to sample size: recruit ment (as discussed above) and attrition. As noted in Chapter 2, attritior rates for the three waves of data collection were similar and did no differentially affect clinical outcomes.

Internal Validity

The Project could also have been considered faulty if its interna validity could be challenged. Internal validity refers to the ability to linl the Demonstration to any outcome in a causal manner (i.e., to have confi dence that the Demonstration, and not some other factor, caused an) observed differences between the Demonstration and Comparison sites) Basically, at question is whether the Demonstration caused any positive o: negative outcomes. The most plausible threats to internal validity in thi: study were the initial and subsequent equivalency of the Demonstratior and Comparison samples. These threats are labeled "selection artifacts' and "differential attrition." Any differences between the samples, eithe: initially or at subsequent waves, that could plausibly explain any finding: would have threatened the conclusion that the Demonstration caused th effect.

Because the design was quasi-experimental, it was possible for there to be large initial differences between the participants in the Demonstration and those in the Comparison sample. Moreover, differential attrition in later waves of data collection could have made interpretation of the data difficult. While we attempted to recruit similar clients at the two sites, field staff had to depend on volunteer participants. Chapter 3 and Chapter 6 provided detailed information showing the initial and subsequent equivalency of the Demonstration and Comparison Evaluation Samples. While it is evident that such equivalence existed, every major analysis of outcome still included a test for equivalency at intake on the particular outcome variable studied.

Construct Validity

The Demonstration could not be seen as effective if the wrong outcome measures were chosen or if the measures used were not sensitive enough to detect change. For example, if IQ scores were examined as an important outcome and found to show no changes, then the Project could report that the Demonstration was ineffective. However, since the Demonstration did not target intelligence as an outcome, and the theory of the Demonstration does not predict any changes in IQ, this conclusion would not be fair. Aside from the possibility of selecting the wrong outcome measures, insensitive measures could have been chosen. Poor measurement was, in fact, a realistic possibility, since the field of child and adolescent mental health measurement and evaluation is in its infancy. The problem of measurement is typically labeled as a threat to construct validity (Cook & Shadish, 1994).

It was not likely that inappropriate outcomes were selected. Authorities acting for the Army, the State of North Carolina, and the Demonstration reviewed the targeted outcomes and agreed on their significance. To guard against the danger of selecting inappropriate or insensitive measures, several steps were taken in planning the Project. First, widely used and accepted outcome measures were used. Second, for the most critical outcome (mental health status), multiple measures were obtained from multiple informants. Third, the Evaluation has attempted to validate the instruments on the data collected for the project. For example, as noted earlier, it was found that the measures of psychopathology correlated with the level of care that the clients received.

In the development of the instrument package, each instrument underwent a series of pilot tests and subsequent refinements. Several instruments were adapted for use in this package and altered to eliminate duplication of items among instruments and to enhance readability. The instrument package underwent review by members of a family advocacy organization, as well as by African-American and Hispanic mental health experts, for possible cultural biases.

To assure high-quality interview data, all interviewers participated in an intensive training program and had to reach a criterion level in the administration of the Child Assessment Schedule on five practice cases. To maintain quality, every interview (with the participant's permission) was recorded on either video- or audiotape, and a 10% sample of each interviewer's tapes was reviewed by a trained instructor, with feedback going to both the interviewer and his or her Site Coordinator. Remediation training was required if the interviewer fell below criterion level.

Another way in which construct validity could have been compromised was if, in fact, the Comparison site system of care was equivalent to that of the Demonstration site (i.e., if the Comparison site also provided a continuum of care). However, the Comparison site provided no features found in the continuum model. For example, it had no single point of entry, no comprehensive intake procedure, no multidisciplinary treatment teams, no case management, and no intermediate services. Thus, it is unlikely that the equivalent clinical outcomes found by the Project could be explained by pointing to equivalent systems of care.

Generalizability of the Fort Bragg Demonstration

Meaning of Generalizability

Generalizability, or the external validity of the results of this evaluation, is concerned with whether the results reported herein generalize to other populations of clients and other operationalizations of the theory of a continuum of care (Costner, 1989; Sussmann & Robertson, 1986). To answer this question, three areas need to be examined: (1) the similarity of the continuum care as implemented in the Demonstration to other interventions, (2) the similarity of the client population to other populations that may receive treatment in a continuum of care, and (3) the degree to which client characteristics differentially affect the success of a continuum of care. That is, are certain subgroups of clients differentially affected by a continuum of care?

Similarity of the Fort Bragg Continuum of Care to Other Demonstrations

As noted in Chapter 1, the primary purpose of the Demonstration was to test the theory that a continuum of care will have better clinical outcomes and lower costs per treated case than the usual fragmented way of delivering services. The theory is the focus of this Demonstration. Does this theory apply to other types of interventions currently being implemented in the field and similar ones in the future? Chapter 1 described the studies supported by the Robert Wood Johnson Foundation (RWJF) that examines systems of care interventions. Clearly, the continuum of care is at the heart of the RWJF demonstrations. The service system that was to be developed in each community was a continuum of care, but *before* the continuum could be implemented, it had to be preceded by interagency coordination and, typically, pooling of funds. These initial efforts can be characterized as developing a system of care in contrast to a continuum of care. Thus, the RWJF provided funds for interagency efforts and case management, but not for the actual continuum-of-care services. The assumption was made that if the system of care was successfully implemented, then a continuum of care would follow. The results of the evaluation of the adult demonstration did not support this assumption. A continuum of care was not developed in these communities, primarily because of a lack of funds. Thus, the continuum-of-care theory was not even tested in this demonstration.

The Comprehensive Community Mental Health Services Program for Children and Adolescents with Serious Emotional Disturbances (SED), described in Chapter 1, is a mixture of both systems change and continuum of care. In order to receive federal funding, a state had to show that interagency coordination was likely. However, in contrast to the RWJF demonstrations, federal funds were also made available for the continuum-of-care services. For these sites to show positive clinical and cost outcomes, they have to implement successfully *both* a system of care and a continuum of care. The Fort Bragg Demonstration, because of the single funding stream, was required only to implement a continuum of care. Thus, the Fort Bragg Demonstration was both a simpler and a purer test of the continuum-of-care theory.

It should be understood that changes that create systems of care cannot directly affect clinical outcomes. An interagency agreement will not improve clinical outcomes for children unless the children receive some services that they would not have received had there not been a change at the system level. That is, system-of-care clinical effects are mediated through the services that children receive. The service model in all current system changes is a managed continuum of care like the one implemented at Fort Bragg.

This flow model can be represented graphically as follows:

System change → Continuum of care → Clinical outcomes

Similarity of Children Treated at Fort Bragg
to Other Treated Children

The data in Chapter 3 suggest that the children who participated in the Evaluation were similar to children in the civilian sector. In general, they are similar to most middle and lower middle class children and adolescents in treatment. However, the Demonstration differs in a major way from projects implemented in the RWJF Mental Health Services for Youth and services funded through the Center for Mental Health Services Comprehensive Community Mental Health Services Program for Children and Adolescents with SED. These programs deal primarily with poor, publicly funded children from multiproblem families. The Demonstration's children were primarily from two-parent families, with good education and middle to lower incomes. Thus, one must raise the question whether the continuum of care would operate the same way with children who were from more impoverished environments.

Interactions between the Continuum and Client Characteristics

This aspect of the discussion focuses on the question whether the continuum would be differentially effective with different types of clients. On the one hand, it could be argued that the complexity of the continuum and its demands on the primary caretaker's time and commitment may also make it more difficult for multiple-problem, low-socioeconomic-status (SES) families to stay in treatment. On the other hand, it can be reasoned that a continuum would be more effective with these families because it would provide the support that they need to receive and stay in services. Both points of view have merit. The inability to clearly understand how client characteristics would operate in a continuum underlines some of the vagueness of the continuum-of-care theory. Unquestionably, much more thought and effort need to be expended in developing and specifying this theory.

In Chapter 5, the effectiveness of the continuum on mental health outcomes was compared for multiproblem families and for the SES and demographic characteristics of clients. None of these variables modified the overall conclusion that the continuum produced effects similar to those produced by the services provided at the Comparison site. While these results cannot be taken as definitive, since the lowest-income families were not present in the study, there were no findings that indicated that a continuum of care would be more effective with different subgroups of clients or families.

The findings of the Fort Bragg Evaluation indicate that the Demonstration provided the *optimal* conditions under which to test a continuum-of-care theory. As Palumbo and Oliverio (1989, p. 342) note, "The concern of external validity is generalizing to *future* applications. In doing this, we should be concerned with whether a better program can be put into place in future locations." It is highly unlikely that a continuum of care, in the present or in the future, will have the extensive financial and human resources that the Demonstration had. If the continuum was not successful under these conditions (i.e., abundant funds, minimal interagency problems, intact families), then it is unlikely to be more successful under more difficult conditions.

SUMMARY OF IMPLEMENTATION ISSUES

In summary, it should be clear that many assumptions underlie the seemingly simple concept of a continuum of care. In order for the continuum to positively affect the lives of children, the service system must satisfy several difficult criteria. It must implement the system with great fidelity and use system-level interventions (e.g., case management) of unknown but assumed effectiveness, and it must deliver services in community settings with the belief that these services are clinically effective. These tasks require multifaceted skills and are difficult to accomplish. If these complex tasks are accomplished, then evaluation methods must also be valid and meet critical assumptions. Strong evidence has been presented that these challenges were met. The evidence is very clear that the Demonstration and the Project were properly implemented; they provided the proper test of the theory of a continuum of care. What, then, are the conclusions that can be drawn from this study?

IMPLICATIONS AND CONCLUSIONS

The Demonstration increased access for children, and those were the children it was appropriate to treat. It is widely recognized that the children in this country are underserved with respect to mental health services. It is estimated that about 2% of the child population receives mental health services (Burns, 1991). Best estimates are that 12–18% of all children require services. At the Comparison site, the typical CHAMPUS system provided care to about 2.7% of all children. The addition of Gateway appears to have improved access to outpatient services to 4.5% at Fort Campbell in fiscal year 1993, in contrast to 8% for that year at the Demonstration site. On the basis of these data, it is clear that the military is providing greater access to mental health services than that found in the general population. However, the Demonstration vastly improved access.

The Demonstration tripled the percentage of eligible children treated in its catchment area. The exact cause of this increase is difficult to determine, as a number of factors changed simultaneously. The Rumbaugh Clinic created a great deal of community awareness about the availability of care and most likely helped reduce the stigma associated with mental health treatment. In addition, lack of a financial barrier was important in motivating parents to bring their children to treatment. Finally, the speed with which clients were treated helped increase satisfaction with the intake and assessment process.

The Project provides important information concerning the appropriateness of accepting these "new" children into treatment. Children at both sites met the Project's independent assessment of a diagnosable mental illness. Over 85% of the children had a moderate or severe functional impairment. The need for these children to receive services was also validated independently by an Army child psychiatrist. Thus, children at both sites required treatment, but the Demonstration treated three times as many children.

The Demonstration successfully implemented a continuum of care. There has been much discussion among mental health experts about the desirability of a continuum of care, yet none was ever implemented on a large scale before the Fort Bragg Demonstration. As discussed throughout this book, Demonstration leadership and staff implemented a program that maintained excellent fidelity to its model. This book, and the previous Quality and Implementation Study reports, have provided considerable evidence that the Demonstration was an excellent representation of the model. The development and implementation of the model are the outstanding contributions of the Demonstration. This accomplishment stands in contrast to other demonstrations of system change (described in Chapter 1).

Implementation was easier to accomplish at the Demonstration site for several reasons. First, a single agency provided or managed all the services; there were few difficulties in coordinating services with other agencies. Second, the Demonstration was funded by one source (unlike, for example, demonstrations that required long negotiations among multiple agencies and funding sources). Third, the Demonstration was very well funded; in other studies the lack of clinical effects were attributed to the unavailability of funds for services. Thus, the full program model in those studies could not be tested because of a shortage of appropriate services. This book amply demonstrates that sufficient services were made available to Demonstration children in need. Thus, lack of differential outcomes was not caused by a shortfall in the availability of services.

The Demonstration successfully treated children in less restrictive environments. Before the Demonstration was implemented, there was concern that not hospitalizing children or not placing them in RTCs may have adverse effects on them. It had never been demonstrated that an extensive continuum of care that placed children in less restrictive settings would not harm children as some feared. Results of the Demonstration clearly indicate that no adverse effects were associated with the use of less restrictive environments.

Parents and adolescents were more satisfied. Extensive data were collected on satisfaction of adolescents and parents with services. While both sites showed satisfaction with services, the Demonstration showed even greater satisfaction. Greatest satisfaction was expressed about services unique to the continuum-of-care model.

Cost control through appropriate care was not demonstrated to be effective. As noted in Chapter 1, another theory tested in this evaluation was the manner in which costs were to be controlled. The Demonstration was under contract to provide services on a cost-reimbursement basis. If costs rose beyond those expected, as they did, the contractor was not responsible (as long as the services were therapeutically appropriate). Most other models of managed care include some shared risk between the provider and the funder. Here, the Army was responsible for paying for all increased costs.

The theory of cost control tested in the Demonstration was that clinicians and their managers, by placing children in the least restrictive and most appropriate level of care, would save money because more expensive and restrictive services would not have to be used. This clinical judgement model proved not to be cost-effective. Costs per client were substantially higher at the Demonstration site. As noted in Chapter 7, these higher costs were primarily related to longer treatment and the use of more expensive intermediate level services, without a significant reduction in the use of the traditional services (i.e., outpatient, hospital, and RTC).

It is also likely that decisions to terminate treatment are difficult for clinicians to make. No research-based guidelines or protocols in the treatment of children exist that would aid in this decision-making process. In the face of this lack of information, caps on service use represent an attempt to provide standardized termination practices.

A continuum of care is not necessarily more expensive. Although costs per treated child were substantially higher at the Demonstration site, it should not necessarily be concluded that a continuum of care is more expensive than other treatment systems. As noted above, the funding of the Demonstration as a cost-reimbursement contract was probably more responsible for the lack of cost control than any features of the continuum. The Demonstration was not designed to control costs through the limitation of services. Rather, the Demonstration focused on reducing hospital-based treatment and testing intermediate services in its place. The management of the Rumbaugh Clinic was not told by the Army to try to control costs through utilization review until January 1994. Thus, it would be inaccurate to attribute the added costs of the Demonstration solely to the continuum.

Although the Demonstration and its Evaluation Project were well implemented, they still had limitations. The cost of not providing services to children at the Comparison site is unknown. We had no information on how many children were placed in detention facilities or required special education. Between-site comparisons could not include the costs to society of not treating children. It was possible, however, to determine how large those costs would have had to be in order to explain the between-site differences. This was done by first calculating the number of children that would have been treated at the Comparison site had access been equal (in other words, had the percentage of eligible children been equivalent). If 13.58% of eligible children had been treated during the Demonstration period at the Comparison site, an additional 2861 children would have received services. To explain the over $33 million difference in costs between sites, these children would have to have imposed an average cost on society of $11,634 each over the 3-year Demonstration period. This example helps make concrete what these costs would have to have been in order for the sites to be equal. Is it reasonable to assume that the untreated children at the Comparison site would have cost society approximately $3878 per year in other costs? This cost is higher than that experienced for the treated children. No published research helps answer questions about whether mental health treatment, for this population, would avoid these costs.

Lack of clinical differences in outcomes leads to questions about current clinical practices. To some, the single most surprising finding of the Project will be the lack of differences in clinical outcomes between the Demonstration and Comparison sites. The failure to find such differences raises a number of concerns. As discussed earlier, the findings argue *against* interpreting these results as caused by poor program implementation, an equivalent system existing at the Comparison site, or an inadequate evaluation. It is thus puzzling that a system of care containing all the features that most experts believe are important determinants of clinical outcomes should show no enhanced clinical effects and furthermore be more costly.

This evaluation brings into question currently held beliefs among experts concerning the necessity for a continuum of care and many of its features. It has been shown that the Demonstration had a more systematic and comprehensive assessment and treatment planning approach, more parent involvement, better case management, more individualized services, fewer treatment dropouts, a greater range of services, enhanced continuity of care, increased length of treatment, and better match between treatment and needs as judged by parents. Still, there were no better outcomes reported. Thus, commonly accepted wisdom about what is a better-quality system of care is called into question. A fragmented system of care, without these features, performed as well in this evaluation.

The alternative to considering the continuum-of-care model unsuccessful is to challenge the assumption that clinical services provided in the community are effective. However, the Project was not designed to examine this question. Children at both sites improved significantly. While it is possible that all this improvement was due to statistical artifacts (e.g., regression to the mean) or spontaneous recovery, it is plausible that treatment had a positive effect at both sites. However, it should be noted that there are fewer than ten scientifically credible studies in the research literature that examine psychotherapy in community settings. These studies, on average, found no effect when treated children were compared to an untreated group of children. This is in contrast to hundreds of studies of psychotherapy in research settings that demonstrated significant and clinically meaningful effects. It is clear that this issue is in need of much more study.

It is also important to stress that clinical outcomes were studied by the Project for only 1 year after children entered the study. We have received additional support from the National Institute of Mental Health to follow the participants in the Outcome Study for 3 more years. This longer time perspective may reveal differences between the sites that we could not find in only 1 year of data collection.

References

Achenbach, T. M. (1991). *Manual for the Child Behavior Checklist and 1991 Profile.* Burlington: University of Vermont Department of Psychiatry.

Achenbach, T. M., & Edelbrock, C. (1983). *Manual for the Child Behavior Checklist and revised Child Behavior Profile.* Burlington: University of Vermont Department of Psychiatry.

Achenbach, T. M., & Edelbrock, C. (1987). *Manual for the Youth Self-Report and Profile.* Burlington: University of Vermont Department of Psychiatry.

American Psychiatric Association. (1987). *Diagnostic and statistical manual of mental disorders,* 3rd ed.—revised. Washington, DC: American Psychiatric Association.

American Psychological Association Practice Directorate (1992). Integrated care challenges managed care. *Practitioner, 5*(2), 1.

Bachrach, L. L. (1980). Is the least restrictive environment always the best: Sociological and semantic implications. *Hospital and Community Psychiatry, 31*(2), 97–103.

Bachrach, L. L. (1981). Continuity of care for chronic mental patients: A conceptual analysis. *American Journal of Psychiatry, 138*(11), 1449–1455.

Baine, D. P. (1992). Prepared statement to the select committee on children, youth and families of the United States House of Representatives. In *The profits of misery: How inpatient psychiatric treatment bilks the system and betrays our trust (GPO 1992-52-362).* Washington, DC: U.S. Government Printing Office.

Banspach, S. W. (1986). *An investigation of three theoretical models of parental satisfaction with early intervention programs for handicapped preschoolers.* Unpublished doctoral dissertation. Nashville: Peabody College of Vanderbilt University.

Behar, L. (1985). Changing patterns of state responsibility: A case study of North Carolina. Special issue: Mental health services to children. *Journal of Clinical Child Psychology, 14*(3), 188–195.

Behar, L. (1992). A need for public academic collaboration in the training of child mental health professionals. In P. Wohlford (Ed.), *CASSP/NIMH Conference Proceedings on Public–Academic Linkage.* Washington, DC: CASSP Technical Assistance Center, Georgetown University.

Behar, L., Bickman, L., Lane, T., Keeton, W. P., & Schwartz, M. (1995). Fort Bragg Child and Adolescent Mental Health Demonstration Project. In N. Roberts (Ed.), *Model practices in service delivery in child and family mental health.* Hillsdale, NJ: Erlbaum Associates (in press).

Berwick, D. M. (1990). *Curing health care: New strategies for quality improvement*. San Francisco: Jossey-Bass.

Bickman, L. (1985). Improving established statewide programs: A component theory of evaluation. *Evaluation Review, 9*, 189–208.

Bickman, L. (Ed.) (1987). *Using program theory in evaluation*. San Francisco: Jossey-Bass.

Bickman, L. (Ed.). (1990). *Advances in program theory*. San Francisco: Jossey-Bass.

Bickman, L. (1992). Designing outcome evaluations for children's mental health services: Improving internal validity. In L. Bickman & D. J. Rog (Eds.), *Evaluating mental health services for children: New directions for program evaluation, 54* (pp. 57–68). San Francisco: Jossey-Bass.

Bickman, L., Bryant, D., & Summerfelt, T. (1993). *Final report of the Quality Study of the Fort Bragg Evaluation Project*. Unpublished manuscript. Nashville: Vanderbilt University Center for Mental Health Policy.

Bickman, L., & Dokecki, P. (1989). The for-profit delivery of mental health services. *American Psychologist, 44*(8), 1133–1137.

Bickman, L., Heflinger, C., Pion, G., & Behar, L. (1992). Evaluation planning for an innovative children's mental health system. *Clinical Psychology Review, 12*(8), 853–865.

Bickman, L., & Peterson, K. (1990). Using program theory to describe and measure program quality. In L. Bickman (Ed.), *Advances in program theory* (pp. 61–72). San Francisco: Jossey-Bass.

Bickman, L., & Rog, D. J. (1995). *Children's mental health services: Research, policy, and innovation*. In L. Bickman & D. J. Rog (Eds.), *Children's mental health services*, Vol. 1. Newbury Park, CA: Sage Publications.

Brandenburg, N. A., Friedman, R., & Silver, S. E. (1990). The epidemiology of childhood psychiatric disorders: Prevalence findings from recent studies. *Journal of the American Academy of Child and Adolescent Psychiatry, 29*, 76–83.

Brannan, A. M., Heflinger, C. A., & Bickman, L. (1994). *Validating the Burden of Care Questionnaire*. Unpublished manuscript. Nashville: Vanderbilt University.

Brown, L., Cox, G. B., Jones, W. E., Semke, J., Allen, D. G., Gilchrist, L. D., & Sutphen-Mroz, J. (1994). Effects of mental health reform on client characteristics, continuity of care, and community tenure. *Evaluation and Program Planning, 17*(1), 63–72.

Bryk, A. S., Raudenbush, S. W., & Congdon, R. T. (1994). *HLM23: Hierarchical linear modeling with the HLM/2L and HLM/3L programs*. Chicago Scientific Software International.

Burchard, J. D., & Schaefer, M. (1992). Improving accountability in a service delivery system in children's mental health. *Clinical Psychology Review, 12*, 867–882.

Burns, B. J. (1991). Mental health service use by adolescents in the 1970s and 1980s. *Journal of the Academy of Child and Adolescent Psychiatry, 30*(1), 144–150.

Burns, B. (1994). The challenges of child mental health services research. *Journal of Emotional and Behavioral Disorders, 2*, 254–259.

Capaldi, D., & Patterson, G. R. (1987). An approach to the problem of recruitment and retention rates for longitudinal research. *Behavioral Assessment, 9*, 169–177.

Cardinal Mental Health Group. (1990a). *Rumbaugh Clinic intake/assessment procedures*. Unpublished manuscript. Fayetteville, NC.

Cardinal Mental Health Group. (1990b). *Treatment philosophy*. Unpublished manuscript. Fayetteville, NC.

Carpenter, M. D. (1978). Residential placement for the chronic psychiatric patient: A review and evaluation of the literature. *Schizophrenia Bulletin, 4*(3), 384–398.

Casey, R. J., & Berman, J. S. (1985). The outcome of psychotherapy with children. *Psychological Bulletin, 98*, 388–400.

Chen, H. (1990). *Theory-driven evaluations*. Newbury Park, CA: Sage Publications.

Chen, H., & Rossi, P. H. (1983). Evaluating with sense: The theory driven approach. *Evaluation Review, 7,* 283–302.

Chen, H., & Rossi, P. H. (1992). *Using theory to improve program and policy evaluation.* New York: Greenwood Press.

Cohen, R., Singh, N. N., Hosick, J., & Tremaine, L. (1992). Implementing a responsive system of mental health services for children. *Clinical Psychology Review, 12,* 819–828.

Cole, R. F., & Poe, S. L. (1993). *Partnerships for care: Systems of care for children with serious emotional disturbances and their families.* Washington, DC: Washington Business Group on Health.

Cook, T., & Shadish, W. (1994). Social experiments: Some developments over the past fifteen years. *Annual Review of Psychology, 45,* 545–580.

Costello, E. J. (1989). Developments in child psychiatric epidemiology. *Journal of the American Academy of Child and Adolescent Psychiatry, 28,* 836–841.

Costner, H. (1989). The validity of conclusions in evaluation research: A further develpment of Chen & Rossi's theory-driven approach. *Evaluation & Program Planning, 12*(4), 345–353.

Coulam, R. F., Smith, J. C. H., Thompson, J. W., Goldman, H. H., Burns, B. J., & Berg, R. F. (1990). *Evaluation of the CPA—Norfolk demonstration: Final report.* Cambridge: Abt Associates.

Cowen, E. L. (1980). The Primary Mental Health Project: Yesterday, today and tomorrow. *Journal of Special Education, 14,* 133–154.

Cronbach, L. J., & Furby, L. (1970). How should we measure change—or should we? *Psychological Bulletin, 74,* 68–80.

Davis, M., Yelton, S., & Katz-Leavy, J. (1993). Unclaimed children revisited: The status of children's mental health services. In C. J. Liberton, K. Kutash, & R. Friedman (Eds.), *Sixth annual research conference proceedings: A system of care for children's mental health: Expanding the research base* (pp. 121–129). Tampa: Research and Training Center for Children's Mental Health, Florida Mental Health Institute.

Dorken, H. (1977). CHAMPUS ten-state claim experience for mental disorder: Fiscal year 1975. *American Psychologist, 32*(9), 697–710.

Dorken, H., VandenBos, G. R., Cummings, N., & Pallak, M. (1993). Impact of law and regulation on professional practice and use of mental health services: An empirical analysis. *Professional Psychology: Research and Practice, 24*(3), 256–265.

Dorwart, R. A., Schelsinger, M., Davidson, H., Epstein, S., & Hoover, P. (1991). A national study of psychiatric hospital care. *American Journal of Psychiatry, 148*(2), 204–210.

Dryfoos, J. (1990). *Adolescents at risk: Prevalence and prevention.* New York: Oxford University Press.

Dunst, C. J. (1986a). *A short form scale for measuring parental health and well-being.* Unpublished manuscript.

Dunst, C. J. (1986b). *Measuring parent commitment to professionally prescribed, child-level interventions.* Unpublished manuscript.

Dunst, C. J., & Leet, H. E. (1987). Measuring the adequacy of resources in households with young children. *Child: Care, Health and Development, 13,* 111–125.

Durenberger, D., & Foote, S. (1993). Beyond incrementalism: Defining and infrastructure for reform. *American Psychologist, 48*(3), 277–282.

Edelbrock, C., & Achenbach, T. (1984). The teacher version of the Child Behavior Profile: I. Boys aged 6–11. *Journal of Consulting and Clinical Psychology, 52,* 207–217.

Elliott, D. S., Huizinga, D., & Menard, S. (1989). *Multiple problem youth: Delinquency, substance use, and mental health problems.* New York: Springer-Verlag.

Endicott, J., Spitzer, R. L., Fleiss, J. L., & Cohen, J. (1976). The Global Assessment Scale: A procedure for measuring overall severity of psychiatric disturbance. *Archives of General Psychiatry, 33,* 766–771.

Epstein, N. B., Baldwin, L. M., & Bishop, D. S. (1983). The McMaster Family Assessment Device. *Journal of Marital and Family Therapy, 9,* 171–180.

Fagan, J. (1991). Community-based treatment for mentally disordered juvenile offenders. *Journal of Clinical Child Psychology, 20,* 42–50.

Fernandez-Pol, B. (1988). Does the military family syndrome exist? *Military Medicine, 153*(8), 418–420.

Flannery, D. (1992). *Report of the review of the quality assurance mechanisms at the Fort Bragg Child and Adolescent Mental Health Demonstration.* Unpublished manuscript, October 1992. San Antonio: U.S. Army Health Services Command.

Folland, S., Goodman, A. C., & Stano, M. (1993). *The economics of health and health care.* New York: Macmillan.

Fowler, W., Keeler, E., & Keesey, J. (1981). *Rand note: The episodes-of-illness processing system.* Santa Monica, CA: Rand.

Frank, R. G., & Dewa, C. S. (1992). Insurance, system structure, and the use of mental health services by children and adolescents. *Clinical Psychology Review, 12,* 829–840.

Friedman, R., & Kutash, K. (1992). Challenges for child and adolescent mental health. *Health Affairs, 1,* 125–136.

Furey, W., & Basili, L. (1988). Predicting satisfaction in parent training for noncompliant children. *Behavior Therapy, 19,* 555–564.

General Accounting Office (1992). *Defense health care: CHAMPUS Mental Health Demonstration Project in Virginia (GAO/HRD 95-93).* Washington, DC: General Accounting Office.

General Accounting Office (1993a). *Defense health care: Additional improvements needed in CHAMPUS' mental health program (GAO/HRD 93-94).* Washington, DC: General Accounting Office.

General Accounting Office (1993b). *Psychiatric fraud and abuse: Increased scrutiny of hospital stays is needed for federal health programs (GAO/HRD 93-92).* Washington, DC: General Accounting Office.

General Accounting Office (1993c). *Managed health care: Effect on employers' costs difficult to measure (GAO/HRD 94-3).* Washington, DC: General Accounting Office.

Gesten, E. (1976). A Health Resources Inventory: The development of a measure of the personal and social competence of primary grade children. *Journal of Consulting and Clinical Psychology, 44,* 775–786.

Goldman, H. H., Morrissey, J. P., & Ridgely, S. M. (1994). Evaluating the Robert Wood Johnson Foundation program on chronic mental illness. *Milbank Quarterly, 72*(1), 37–48.

Goldman, H. H., Scheffler, R. M., & Cheadle, A. (1987). Demand for psychiatric services: A clinical episode model for specifying "the product." *Advances in Health Economics and Health Services Research, 8,* 255–273.

Grad, J., & Sainsbury, P. (1968). The effects that patients have on their families in a community care and a control psychiatric service—a two year follow up. *British Journal of Psychiatry, 114*(508), 265–278.

Gramlich, E. M. (1981). *Benefit–cost analysis of government programs.* Englewood Cliffs, NJ: Prentice-Hall.

Haas-Wilson, D., Cheadle, A., & Scheffler, R. (1989). Demand for mental health services: An episode of treatment approach. *Southern Economic Journal, 56*(1), 219–232.

Haberken, R. C. (1991). Letter to Lenore Behar (regarding review at Rumbaugh completed August 6, 1991, and September 10, 1991), Sept. 16, Winston-Salem, NC: Forsyth-Stokes area MH/DD/SA Program.

Harnett, D. L. (1980). *Introductory statistical analysis.* Reading, MA: Addison-Wesley.

Harter, S. (1982). The Perceived Competence Scale for Children. *Child Development, 53,* 87–97.

Harter, S. (1985). *Manual for the Self-Perception Profile for Children.* Denver: University of Denver Press.

Hedrick, T., Bickman, L., & Rog, D. (1993). *Planning applied social research.* Newbury Park, CA: Sage Publications.

Heflinger, C. (1993). *Final report of Fort Bragg Evaluation: The Implementation Study.* Unpublished manuscript. Nashville: Vanderbilt University Center for Mental Health Policy.

Herjanic, B., Herjanic, M., Brown, F., & Wheatt, T. (1975). Are children reliable reporters? *Journal of Abnormal Child Psychology, 3*(1), 41–48.

Herjanic, B., & Reich, W. (1982). Development of a structured psychiatric interview for children: Agreement between child and parent on individual symptoms. *Journal of Abnormal Child Psychology, 10*(3), 307–324.

Hightower, A. D., Work, W. C., Cowen, E. L., Lotyczewski, B., Spinell, A. P., Guare, J. C., & Rohrbeck, C. A. (1986). The Teacher–Child Rating Scale: A brief objective measure of elementary children's school problem behaviors and competencies. *School Psychology Review, 15*(3), 393–409.

Hobbs, N. (1982). *The troubled and troubling child.* San Francisco: Jossey-Bass.

Hodges, K. (1990). *The Child and Adolescent Functional Assessment Scale (CAFAS).* Unpublished manuscript.

Hodges, K., Bickman, L., Ring-Kurtz, S., & Reiter, M. (1992). A multi-dimensional measure of level of functioning in children and adolescents. In A. Algarin & R. Friedman (Eds.), *The fourth annual research conference: A system of care for children's mental health: Building a research base* (pp. 149–154). Tampa: Research and Training Center for Children's Mental Health, Florida Mental Health Institute.

Hodges, K., & Cools, J. (1990). Structured diagnostic interviews. In A. M. LaGreca (Ed.), *Through the eyes of the child: Obtaining self-report from children and adolescents* (pp. 109–149). Boston: Allyn & Bacon.

Hodges, K., Kline, J., Stern, L., Cytryn, L., & McKnew, D. (1982). The development of a child assessment interview for research and clinical use. *Journal of Abnormal Child Psychology, 10,* 173–189.

Hodges, K., & Saunders, W. (1989). Internal consistency of a diagnostic interview for children:bThe Child Assessment Schedule (CAS). *Journal of Abnormal Child Psychology, 17,* 691–701.

Hoenig, J., & Hamilton, M. W. (1967). The burden on the household in an extramural psychiatric service. In H. Freeman & M. W. Hamilton (Eds.), *New aspects in mental health services* (pp. 612–635). London: Pergamon Press.

Hornbrook, M. C., Hurtado, A. V., & Johnson, R. E. (1985). Health care episodes: Definition, measurement, and use. *Medical Care Review, 42*(2), 163–218.

Hostetter, R. E. (1994). *Review of Quality Improvement (QI) program.* Unpublished manuscript.

Inouye, S. (1988). Children's mental health issues. *American Psychologist, 43*(10), 813–816.

Interim Report of the Fort Bragg Evaluation Project. (1991). Unpublished manuscript. Nashville: Vanderbilt University Center for Mental Health Policy, April.

Jacobson, N. S., & Truax, P. (1991). Clinical significance: A statistical approach to defining meaningful change in psychopathology research. *Journal of Consulting and Clinical Psychology, 59*(1), 12–19.

JCAHO (Joint Commission on Accreditation of Health Care Organizations) (1991). *Consolidated standards manual.* Oakbrook, IL: JCAHO.

JCAHO (Joint Commission on Accreditation of Health Care Organizations) (1993). *Mental health accreditation manual.* Oakbrook, IL: JCAHO.

Jensen, D. S., Grogan, D., Xenakis, S. N., & Bain, M. W. (1989). Father absence: Effects on child and maternal psychopathology. *Journal of American Academy of Child and Adolescent Psychiatry, 28*(2), 171–175.

Jensen, P. S., Xenakis, S. N., Wolf, P., & Bain, M. W. (1991). The "military family syndrome" revisited: By the numbers. *Journal of Nervous and Mental Disease, 179*, 102–107.

Kalman, T. (1983). An overview of parent satisfaction with psychiatric treatment. *Hospital and Community Psychiatry, 24*, 437–441.

Kashani, J. H., Orvaschel, H., Rosenberg, T., & Reid, J. (1989). Psychopathology among a community sample of children and adolescents: A developmental perspective. *Journal of the American Academy of Child and Adolescent Psychiatry, 28*(5), 701–706.

Kazdin, A. E. (1980). Acceptability of alternative treatments for deviant child behavior. *Journal of Applied Behavior Analysis, 13*, 259–273.

Kazdin, A. E. (1989). Developmental psychopathology: Current research, issues, and directions. *American Psychologist, 44*(2), 180–187.

Kazdin, A. E., Esveldt-Dawson, K., Unis, A., & Rancurello, M. (1983). Child and parent evaluations of depression and aggression in psychiatric inpatient children. *Journal of Abnormal Child Psychology, 11*(3), 401–413.

Kee, J. E. (1994). Benefit–cost analysis in program evaluation. In J. S. Wholey, H. P. Hatry, & K. E. Newcomer (Eds.), *Handbook of practical program evaluation* (pp. 456–488). San Francisco: Jossey-Bass.

Kessler, L. G., Steinwachs, D. M., & Hankin, J. R. (1980). Episodes of psychiatric utilization. *Medical Care, 18*, 1219–1227.

Kiesler, C. A. (1992). U.S. mental health policy: Doomed to fail. *American Psychologist, 47*(9), 1077–1082.

Kiesler, C. A., & Simpkins, C. G. (1991). The de facto national system of psychiatric inpatient care. *American Psychologist, 46*, 579–584.

Kiesler, C. A., & Simpkins, C. G. (1993). *The unnoticed majority in psychiatric inpatient care.* New York: Plenum Press.

Knitzer, J. (1982). *Unclaimed children.* Washington, DC: Children's Defense Fund.

Knitzer, J. (1993). Children's mental health policy: Challenging the future. *Journal of Emotional and Behavioral Disorders, 1*, 8–16.

LaGrone, D. A. (1978). The military family syndrome. *American Journal of Psychiatry, 135*, 1040–1043.

Lambert, E. W. (1993). Monte Carlo modeling. In L. Bickman (Ed.), Response to the directorate of health care studies and clinical investigations final report (revised). Unpublished manuscript. Nashville: Vanderbilt University Center for Mental Health Policy.

Lampman, C., Durlak, J., & Wells, A. (1991). *Statistical power in child psychotherapy research.* Chicago: Loyola University.

Larsen, D., Attkisson, C., Hargreaves, W., & Nguyen, T. (1979). Assessment of client/patient satisfaction in human service programs: Development of a general scale. *Evaluation and Program Planning, 6*, 211–236.

Leaf, P. J., & Bruce, M. L. (1987). Gender differences in the use of mental health–related services: A re-examination. *Journal of Health and Social Behavior, 28*, 171–183.

Lebow, J. (1987). Acceptability as a simple measure in mental health program evaluation. *Evaluation and Program Planning, 10*, 191–195.

Lehman, A. E., Postrado, L. T., Roth, D., McNary, S. W., & Goldman, H. H. (1994). Continuity of care and client outcomes in the Robert Wood Johnson Foundation program on chronic mental illness. *Milbank Quarterly, 72*(1), 105–122.

Lipsey, M. W. (1990). *Design sensitivity.* Newbury Park, CA: Sage Publications.

Lipsey, M. W., Crosse, S., Dunkle, J., Pollard, J., & Stobart, G. (1985). Evaluation: The state of the art and the sorry state of the science. In D. S. Cordray (Ed.), *Utilizing prior research in evaluation planning: New directions for program evaluation 27*, (pp. 7–28). San Francisco: Jossey-Bass.

Lipsey, M. W., & Wilson, D. (1993). The efficacy of psychological, educational, and behavioral treatment. *American Psychologist, 48*(12), 1181–1209.

Lorion, R. P., Cowen, E. L., & Caldwell, R. A. (1975). Normative and parametric analyses of school maladjustment. *American Journal of Community Psychology, 3*, 291–301.

Maloy, K. (1994). *The children's plan*. Unpublished manuscript. Nashville: Vanderbilt University Center for Mental Health Policy, August.

Marchant, K. H., & Medway, F. J. (1987). Adjustment and achievement associated with mobility in military families, *Psychology in the Schools, 24*(3), 289–294.

Martin, E. (1992). Prepared statement to the Select Committee on Children, Youth, and Families, United States House of Representatives. In *The profits of misery: How inpatient psychiatric treatment bilks the system and betrays our trust (GPO 1992-52-362)* (pp. 215–249). Washington, DC: U.S. Government Printing Office.

Maxwell, S. E., & Delaney, H. D. (1993). Bivariate median splits and spurious statistical significance. *Psychological Bulletin, 113*(1), 181–190.

McCubbin, H. (1987). Family Index of Regenerativity and Adaptation—Military. In H. McCubbin & A. Thompson (Eds.), *Family assessment for research and practice*. Madison: University of Wisconsin.

McCubbin, H., & Patterson, J. M. (1981). *FILE: Family Inventory of Life Events and Changes*. St. Paul: University of Minnesota, Family Social Science.

McCubbin, H., & Patterson, J. (1983). Family transitions: Adaptation to stress. In H. I. McCubbin & C. R. Figley (Eds.), *Stress and the family*, Vol. 1, *Coping with normative transitions* (pp. 5–25). New York: Brunner/Mazel.

McCubbin, H., Patterson, J., & Lavee, Y. (1983). *One thousand Army families: Strengths, coping, and supports*. St. Paul: University of Minnesota, Family Social Science.

McGlynn, E. A., Norquist, G. S., Wells, K. B., Sullivan, G., & Lieberman, R. P. (1988). Quality-of-care research in mental health. *Inquiry, 25*, 157–168.

McGuire, T. G. (1991). Measuring the economic cost of schizophrenia. *Schizophrenia Bulletin, 17*(3), 375–388.

Miller, I. W., Epstein, N. B., Bishop, D. S., & Keitner, G. I. (1985). The McMaster Family Assessment Device: Reliability and validity. *Journal of Marital and Family Therapy, 11*(4), 345–356.

Montgomery, R., Stull, D., & Bagatta, E. (1985). Measurement and analysis of burden. *Research on Aging, 7*(1), 137–152.

Morrison, J. (1981). Rethinking the military family syndrome. *American Journal of Psychiatry, 138*, 354–357.

National Mental Health Association (1989). *Invisible children project*. Prepared by C. Zeigleer-Dendy, Alexandria, Virginia.

Navratil, J. L., Green, S., Loeber, R., & Lahey, B. (1994). Minimizing subject loss in a longitudinal study of deviant behavior. *Journal of Child and Family Studies, 3*(1), 89–106.

Newman, S. J., Reschovsky, J. D., Koneda, K., & Hendrick, A. M. (1994). The effects of independent living on persons with chronic mental illness: An assessment of the Section 8 Certificate Program. *Milbank Quarterly, 72*(1), 171–190.

OCHAMPUS (1992). *CHAMPUS Handbook (1992-675-578)*. Washington, DC: U.S. Government Printing Office.

Oswald, D. P., Singh, N. N., & Ellis, C. R. (1992). The current state of child and adolescent mental health services. *Clinical Psychology Review, 12*, 791–793.

Padgett, D. K., Patrick, C., Burns, B. J., Schlesinger, H., & Cohen, J. (1992). The effect of insurance benefit changes on use of child and adolescent outpatient mental health services. *Medical Care, 31*(2), 96–110.

Palumbo, D. J., & Oliverio, A. (1989). Implementation theory and the theory driven approach to validity. Special issue: The theory-driven perspective. *Evaluation and Program Planning*, 12(4), 337–344.

Pascoe, G., & Attkisson, C. (1983). The evaluation ranking scale: A new methodology for assessing satisfaction. *Evaluation and Program Planning*, 6, 335–347.

Patrick, C., Padgett, D. K., Burns, B., Schlesinger, H. J., & Cohen, J. (1993). Use of inpatient services by a national population: Do benefits make a difference? *Journal of the American Academy of Child and Adolescent Psychiatry*, 32(1), 144–152.

Peterson, K., & Bickman, L. (Eds.). (1992). *Normative theory and program quality in mental health services*. Westwood, MA: Greenwood Press.

Phillips, B., & Edwards, L. (1993). Letter to Lenore Behar (regarding eligibility of services), April 22. Fayetteville, NC: Rumbaugh Mental Health Clinic.

Ranshoff, P., Zachary, R. A., Gaynor, J., & Hargreaves, W. A. (1982). Measuring restrictiveness of psychiatric care. *Hospital and Community Psychiatry*, 33(5), 361–366.

Reich, W., & Welner, Z. (1990). *Interview for children and adolescents (rev.): Child version DICA-R-C (DSM-III-R Version)*. St. Louis: Washington University, Division of Child Psychiatry.

Rice, D. P., Kelman, S., Miller, L. S., & Dunmeyer, S. (1990). *The economic costs of alcohol and drug abuse and mental illness, 1985*. Rockville, MD: U.S. Department of Health and Human Services.

Rivera, V. R., & Kutash, K. (1994). *Components of a system of care: What does the research say?* Tampa: University of South Florida, Florida Mental Health Institute, Research and Training Center for Children's Mental Health.

Roberts, M. C. (1994). Models for service delivery in children's mental health: Common characteristics. *Journal of Clinical Child Psychology*, 23, 212–219.

Rog, D. J. (1992). Child and adolescent mental health services: Evaluation challenges. In L. Bickman & D. J. Rog (Eds.), *Evaluating mental health services for children: New directions for program evaluation*, 54 (pp. 5–16). San Francisco: Jossey-Bass.

Rubin, D. R. (1976). Inference and missing data. *Biometrika*, 63, 581–592.

Ruiz, P. (1993). Access to health care for uninsured Hispanics: Policy recommendation. *Hospital and Community Psychiatry*, 44(10), 958–962.

Runyan, D., Everson, M., Edelsohn, G., Hunter, W., & Coulter, M. (1988). Impact of legal intervention on sexually abused children. *Journal of Pediatrics*, 113, 647–653.

Saxe, L., Cross, T., & Silverman, N. (1988). Children's mental health: The gap between what we know and what we do. *American Psychologist*, 43(10), 800–807.

Saxe, L., Cross, T., Silverman, N., Batchelor, W., & Dougherty, D. (1987). *Children's mental health: Problems and treatment*. Durham, NC: Duke University Press.

Schmitz, C. L., & Gilchrist, L. D. (1991). Developing a community-based care system for seriously emotionally disabled children and youth. *Child and Adolescent Social Work*, 8, 417–430.

Select Committee on Children, Youth, and Families, United States House of Representatives (1992). *The profits of misery: How inpatient psychiatric treatment bilks the system and betrays our trust (GPO1992-58-362)*. Washington, DC: U.S. Government Printing Office.

Shaffer, D., Fisher, P., Piacentini, J., Schwab, C., Stone, M., & Wicks, J. (1989). *Diagnostic Interview Schedule for Children: DISC-2.1C, Child Version*. Unpublished manuscript. New York: New York State Psychiatric Institute, Department of Child and Adolescent Psychiatry.

Shaffer, D., Garland, A., Gould, M., & Fisher, P. (1988). Preventing teenage suicide: A critical review. *Journal of the American Academy of Child and Adolescent Psychiatry*, 27(6), 675–687.

Shaffer, D., Gould, M. S., Brasic, J., Ambrosini, P., Fisher, P., Bird, H., & Aluwhalia, S. (1983). A Children's Global Assessment Scale (CGAS). *Archives of General Psychiatry*, 40, 1228–1231.

Shern, D. L., Wilson, N., & Coen, A. S. (1994). Client outcomes II: Longitudinal client data from the Colorado treatment outcome study. *Milbank Quarterly, 72*(1), 123–148.

Silver, A. A. (1984). Children in classes for the severely emotionally handicapped. *Journal of Developmental and Behavioral Pediatrics, 5,* 49–54.

Soler, M., & Shauffer, C. (1990). Fighting fragmentation: Coordination of services for children and families. *Nebraska Law Review, 69,* 278–297.

Stipak, B. (1980). Using clients to evaluate programs. *Computers, Environment, and Urban Systems, 5*(3/4).

Stroul, B. A. (1994). Systems of care for children and adolescents with emotional disorders: What are the results? *Continuum: Developments in Ambulatory Mental Health Care, 1,* 29–49.

Stroul, B. A., & Friedman, R. (1986). *A system of care for children and youth with severe emotional disturbances,* revised ed. Washington, DC: Georgetown University Child Development Center, CASSP Technical Assistance Center.

Sussmann, M., & Robertson, D. U. (1986). The validity of validity: An analysis of validation study design. *Journal of Applied Psychology, 71*(3), 461–468.

Taube, C. A., & Rupp, A. (1986). The effect of Medicaid on access to ambulatory mental health care for the poor and near poor under 65. *Medical Care, 24*(8), 677–686.

Thompson, E. H., & Doll, W. (1982). The burden of families coping with the mentally ill: An invisible crisis. *Family Relations, 31,* 379–388.

Treiber, F. A., & Mabe, P. A. (1987). Child and parent perceptions of children's psychopathology in psychiatric outpatient children. *Journal of Abnormal Child Psychology, 15*(1), 115–124.

Tsai, S. P., Reedy, S. M., Bernacki, E. J., & Lee, E. S. (1988). Effect of curtailed insurance benefits on use of mental health care: The Tenneco plan. *Medical Care, 26*(4), 430–440.

VandenBos, G. R. (1993). U.S. mental health policy: Proactive evolution in the midst of health care reform. *American Psychologist, 48*(3),283–290.

Warner, K. E., & Luce, B. R. (1982). *Cost–benefit and cost–effectiveness analysis in health care.* Ann Arbor, MI: Health Administration Press.

Weisner, C., & Schmidt, L. (1992). Gender disparities in treatment for alcohol problems. *JAMA: The Journal of the American Medical Association, 268*(14), 1872–1876.

Weisz, J. R., & Weiss, B. (1987). Effectiveness of psychotherapy with children and adolescents: A meta-analysis for clinicians. *Journal of Consulting and Clinical Psychology, 55,* 542–549.

Weisz, J. R., & Weiss, B. (1993). *Effects of psychotherapy with children and adolescents.* Newbury Park, CA: Sage Publications.

Weithorn, L. A. (1988). Mental hospitalization of troublesome youth: An analysis of skyrocketing admission rates. *Stanford Law Review, 40,* 773–838.

Wells, K. B. (1988). Quality-of-care in mental health: Policy and personal perspectives. *Focus on Mental Health Services Research, 3*(1), 1.

Wells, K. B., Keeler, E., & Manning, W. G. (1990). Patterns of outpatient mental health care over time: Some implications for estimates of demand and for benefit design. *Health Services Research, 24*(6), 773–789.

Wojcik, B. E., Stein, C. R., & Optenberg, S. A. (1993). *Detailed analysis of CHAMPUS per capita mental health expenditures for beneficiaries less than eighteen: Health services command catchment areas fiscal years 1988–1993.* San Antonio: U.S. Army Medical Department Center and School, Ft. Sam Houston, Tri-Service CHAMPUS Statistical Database Project.

World Health Organization (1978). *International classification of diseases,* 9th ed. Geneva: World Health Organization.

Wyatt, R. J., & Clark, K. (1987). Calculating the cost of schizophrenia. *Psychiatric Annals, 17*(9), 586–591.

Yin, R. K. (1986). *Case study research.* Newbury Park, CA: Sage Publications.

Yin, R. K. (1993). *Applications of case study research.* Newbury Park, CA: Sage Publications.

Index